MENOPAUSE YOGA™ AND WELLBEING

A Daily Practice Guide for Perimenopause to Second Spring

PETRA COVENEY

SINGING DRAGON

LONDON AND PHILADELPHIA

First published in Great Britain in 2025 by Singing Dragon,
an imprint of Jessica Kingsley Publishers
Part of John Murray Press

2

Copyright © Petra Coveney 2025
Illustration © Petra Coveney 2025

The information contained in this book is not intended to replace the services
of trained medical professionals or to be a substitute for medical advice.
The complementary therapy described in this book may not be suitable for
everyone to follow. You are advised to consult a doctor before embarking on any
complementary therapy programme and on any matters relating to your health, and
in particular on any matters that may require diagnosis or medical attention.

A CIP catalogue record for this title is available from the
British Library and the Library of Congress

ISBN 978 1 80501 134 7
eISBN 978 1 80501 135 4

Printed and bound in the United States by Integrated Books International

Jessica Kingsley Publishers' policy is to use papers that are natural,
renewable and recyclable products and made from wood grown in
sustainable forests. The logging and manufacturing processes are expected
to conform to the environmental regulations of the country of origin.

Singing Dragon
Carmelite House
50 Victoria Embankment
London EC4Y 0DZ

www.singingdragon.com

John Murray Press
Part of Hodder & Stoughton Limited
An Hachette UK Company

The authorised representative in the EEA is Hachette Ireland,
8 Castlecourt Centre, Dublin 15, D15 XTP3, Ireland (email: info@hbgi.ie)

'A beautiful, empowering guide packed with practical tools to support women through every stage of menopause. These simple yoga practices are a powerful addition to your self-care toolbox – wherever you are in your journey.'

– Lavina Mehta MBE, personal trainer, author of The Feel Good Fix *and founder of Feel Good with Lavina*

'This book is an absolute gift. It doesn't just give you the information every woman deserves to know about perimenopause, menopause, symptoms and HRT, it goes so much deeper. What makes it truly powerful is how it weaves in the role of yoga and simple, sustainable lifestyle practices to help us navigate this season with strength, clarity and grace. The videos are the cherry on top, practical, thoughtful and so easy to follow. This isn't just a book, it's a toolkit for thriving. Congratulations on creating something so needed and so impactful.'

– Sahir Ahmed, menopause coach and speaker, founder of SAE Empower Coaching

'Petra's comprehensive and holistic guide to supporting and celebrating the menopause transition is an invaluable companion to have by your side as you navigate the challenges that face every woman in midlife. Her wisdom and experience shine through as she gifts us her expertly devised menopause yoga programme which has already benefited thousands of women across the globe.'

– Melinda McDougall MSc, MNIMH, medical herbalist

'I'm delighted Petra has created this vital and inclusive collection of thinking and possibilities. All too often, our menopause work focuses only on what is difficult, what is troubling, what a struggle it all might be. And yes, many of us have found the menopause transition a struggle AND there is still a lot we can do for ourselves. Yoga, in all its forms, the philosophy as well as the embodied practice, offers a beautiful support on our path through the transition.'

– Stella Duffy, UKCP reg, MBACP, MUPCA (Accred), GPsyC

'Petra's new book is a beautifully inclusive, nurturing companion for anyone navigating menopause. It's more than yoga – it's breathwork, journaling, expert insights, a guide and real-life stories, all delivered in a tone that invites rather than instructs. Whether you're brand new to yoga or not, this book meets you where you are – with warmth, wisdom and care.'

– Jinty Sheerin, podcaster of Spill The Tea with Womenkind Collective!

by the same author

Menopause Yoga
A Holistic Guide to Supporting Women on their Menopause Journey
Petra Coveney
ISBN 978 1 78775 889 6
eISBN 978 1 78775 890 2

of related interest

Black and Menopausal
Intimate Stories of Navigating the Change
Edited by Yansie Rolston and Yvonne Christie
Foreword by Iya Rev. DeShannon Barnes-Bowens, M.S.
ISBN 978 1 83997 379 6
eISBN 978 1 83997 380 2

Pain is Really Strange
Graphic Medicine
Steve Haines
Art by Sophie Standing
ISBN 978 1 84819 264 5
eISBN 978 0 85701 212 8

This book is dedicated to all the women in a stage of the menopause who shared their feedback and wisdom, and who trusted me with their personal stories. I hope it becomes your friendly bedside companion to dip into whenever you need. Use it to tune in to what you need, listen to your own wisdom, trust yourself, and make your own self-care a radical act of kindness. Ultimately, I hope it helps you to step into your Second Spring so you can blossom and feel stronger, stable, louder and bolder. We are a generation of women who are not settling for less and we deserve to be heard. Watch out world – we're coming!

About the author

Petra Coveney is a senior yoga teacher, teacher trainer, yoga therapist and founder of Menopause Yoga and the Menopause Yoga and Wellbeing programme (2013).[*] She works with yoga and medical professionals, and was the first yoga teacher to become a member of the British, American and Australasian Menopause societies. She is a yoga advisor to The Menopause Charity and University College London's InTune National Menopause Education and Support Programme. Her Menopause in the Workplace webinars are delivered to international companies and public sector organizations.

Petra launched the first Menopause Yoga teachers' training course in 2019, which is accompanied by her first book, *Menopause Yoga: A Holistic Guide to Supporting Women on their Menopause Journey* (Singing Dragon, 2021). There are currently over 1000 Menopause Yoga-trained teachers in 50 countries, and her course has been translated into Japanese.

As a former BBC radio and television producer, Petra enjoys writing blogs and articles about the menopause for magazines, and is a regular guest on podcasts.

Petra is a mother of two awesome adults and lives with her dog Alfie by the sea in Brighton, East Sussex, where she swims in the sea (almost) every day with the Salty Seabirds.

Menopause Yoga is a UK-registered trademarked name and the visual content is sole property of the creator Petra Coveney.

---

[*]   www.menopause-yoga.com

Acknowledgements

I would like to thank these menopause specialists: Dr Claire Phipps, Dr Radhika Vohra, Simona Stokes, Melinda McDougall and Emma Ellice Flint. Thank you also to these other experts in their field: Professor Joyce Harper, Stella Duffy, Adele Wimsett, Deena Solanki, and Caroline Phipps, who all generously made contributions to this book and are guest speakers on my courses, workshops and retreats. Each of these contributors has a passion for supporting other people in their menopause and beyond. Thank you to poet Noëlle Harrison for her beautiful words.

Thank you to all the women and people who shared their personal stories and provided insights into a diverse range of experiences so that we can all better understand other perspectives: Jinty Sheerin, Patsy Isles, Sarah Thomas, Kat Aydin, Jessica Adams, Caroline Wilkinson, Ayana Williams, and Veronica Santini.

Thank you to forensic illustrator Dr Elysia Greenway and artist David Caines, for their hand-drawn pictures.

Thank you to the Menopause Yoga teachers who feature in the class videos. They are: Razia Sultana, Ayana Williams, Maria Stephens and Zoe Vincent. They all share a commitment to showing real yoga bodies and diversity of representation.

Thank you to filmmaker Sam Morris at Avocado Baby Film for the beautifully composed videos, Sarah Houghton for the photos, and The Brighton Studio for hosting us.

I am indebted to my editor Sarah Hamlin, and publishers Jessica Kingsley Publishers/Singing Dragon for this opportunity to share with you *Menopause Yoga and Wellbeing: A Daily Practice Guide for Perimenopause to Second Spring*.

Contents

Preface: My Story

Perimenopause stopped me in my tracks aged 45. Lost, alone and scared, I felt unsupported and couldn't find reliable self-help information. Back then, the medical term 'menopause' was negatively associated with female decline, infertility, unsympathetic ageing, a descent into social irrelevance. Becoming invisible.

MY STRUGGLE AND SEARCH FOR ANSWERS

My mum had passed away and friends were reluctant to talk, as if mentioning the word 'menopause' would hasten its arrival. Determined not to struggle in silence, I drew on both my yoga teacher training and my BBC journalism background. I scoured the internet for books on menopause nutrition, herbs, supplements, exercise and yoga routines. But the information was scattered, contradictory and overwhelming. I needed a one-stop shop and someone to talk to.

CREATING MY OWN SOLUTION

Shocked by how little information was available, and my own level of ignorance, I sought the medical facts and became the first yoga teacher to join the British Menopause Society (BMS), attending medical menopause conferences and receiving the latest research.

MODIFYING YOGA FOR MENOPAUSE

Traditional yoga texts mostly ignored the menopause because they were written for men, so I experimented by modifying poses and using props to meet my new physical needs in perimenopause. In extreme agony from inflammation causing a frozen shoulder and pain in my lumbar spine, sacroiliac joint and sciatic nerve, I had to learn how to slow down, soften, breathe and find ease in the present moment (sthira, sukham, asanam, Yoga Sutra 2.46).

Gentle somatic movement, water therapy and meditation really helped. Six months later I was pain-free, could touch my toes (an outcome, not the aim) and was smiling with relief. Yoga philosophy helped me accept change and relax instead of resisting menopause.

SELF-COMPASSION

Lifestyle has a huge impact on menopause symptoms. Practising yoga regularly naturally led to my wanting to be healthier, so I stopped wanting to consume wine, coffee and cake. I slept better, had fewer night sweats and felt less fatigued or dehydrated the next day. Most importantly, I learned to love myself more – finally, in my late 40s!

Yoga is rooted in ancient philosophy that recognizes the impermanence and inevitable flow of life. I realized I was afraid of the menopause because it was shrouded in taboo, I was fearful of the future because I lacked information, and my resistance to change was causing physical tension and stress. I had to pause...breathe...let go.

EASTERN INSPIRATION

My mother was half Chinese, so after she passed away, I was drawn to read more about menopause from an Eastern perspective. In Traditional Chinese Medicine (TCM), the post-reproductive stage of life is positively described as a woman's Second Spring, an awakening to herself where her body becomes her own again and she can pursue her own passions and interests (if her children have left home).

In TCM a first sign of menopause is when a woman starts to voice her opinions more strongly, she becomes more authoritative, she steps into her power. As Xiaolan Zhao says in her book *Traditional Chinese Medicine for Women: Reflections of Moon on Water*,[1] a woman steps into wholeness. Wow! This positive perspective completely flipped my negative Western perspective.

At its heart, Menopause Yoga has been designed to be educational and empowering, and to encourage you to embrace this stage of life as an opportunity to step into your Second Spring feeling healthy and happy (see 'Yoga health benefits' in Part Three).

SECOND SPRING

Now, nearly 10 years into my postmenopause, I stand resolutely in my Second Spring, which has shifted into Second Summer, feeling stronger, fitter and confident about how to navigate this incredible journey. Alongside yoga, I also lift weights, swim in the sea, walk my dog and meditate more.

STRENGTH, SELF-LOVE AND RADICAL REST

My body is different today; I love that my muscles feel stronger, but I have more wrinkles on my face and more wobbly bits on my body. Coming through menopause taught me that perfection is overrated and a waste of our precious energy. When I hear that nagging voice of self-doubt, I remember to embrace myself with kindness (my oxytocin hug). Sometimes it also helps to say, 'I don't give a @%*!' This, dear friends, is our menopause superpower.

SHARING MY KNOWLEDGE AND EMPOWERING OTHERS

Since 2013, the success of the Menopause Yoga and Wellbeing programme has been humbling, with women and teachers worldwide joining me in workshops, classes, retreats and training courses. My first book was written to accompany the professionally accredited 40-hour Menopause Yoga teachers' training course. This new book is written specially for women and people, like you, going through perimenopause to postmenopause. It includes simple, short home practices that you can fit into your day and evening.

I hope this book becomes a bedside table friend that you dip into where you are in your menopause journey, which can be 7–10 years or more! Let's make these our best years. The so-called 'change' is not an end, dear friends; it is a wake-up call to the next chapter of your awesome life. Let's educate ourselves, reframe menopause positively, and become role models for the next generation: our sisters, daughters, families, friends, work colleagues and communities.

Menopausal women are a force to be reckoned with – society's movers, shakers, agitators and changemakers as well as friends and carers who may hold the fabric of our families together. Together, let's be the change we want to see in the world.

Watch Petra's welcome message, introducing you to the videos that accompany her book.

Introduction

Yoga isn't a magic pill cure; it is a valuable piece of the holistic healthcare puzzle.

WHY YOGA?

The benefits of a regular yoga practice are well researched and include:

- Reduced stress and inflammation. Yoga can help you manage stress, a common contributor to menopausal symptoms. It can also reduce inflammation in the body, which may ease aches and pains associated with menopause.

- Support for endocrine and digestive systems. By reducing stress and inflammation, yoga postures and breathing exercises may improve digestion and elimination (to counter bloating and constipation), both of which can be affected by oestrogen fluctuations and cortisol during menopause.

- Improved mental and emotional wellbeing. Yoga may enhance your mood, ease anxiety and promote better sleep, all of which contribute to emotional wellbeing during menopause.

- Enhanced balance, muscle tone and spatial awareness. Proprioception, muscle tone and movement coordination can significantly reduce your risk of falls and osteoporotic fractures.

- Developing interoception. Our ability to sense internal physical and emotional states is vital for menopause self-care, allowing us to adjust our daily routines based on how we feel, which can fluctuate wildly in our perimenopause due to hormone instability.

- Complementary therapies. Yoga's unique mind–body approach complements other exercise, nutrition, therapies and medical interventions.

- Gentle place to start. For those feeling unfit, recovering from injury or low physical self-confidence, yoga offers a gentle self-care starting point. It can be a stepping stone to other exercise.

So yoga is *not* a magic cure-all pill, but it is a valuable part of a holistic programme that is recommended by other health professionals.

MAKE YOGA A HABIT

Take a daily dip, learn when you're feeling well, make it part of a daily routine, as a preventative to help you manage stress and alleviate some symptoms. Yoga is not just stretchy poses; it's a holistic practice underpinned by a philosophy that helps you to accept change as inevitable, tune into yourself and inner wisdom, and enjoy the journey.

WHY MENOPAUSE YOGA?

Menopause Yoga aims to educate and empower you by providing specific tools and techniques for alleviating some of the main symptoms, while positively reframing the menopause as your Second Spring. Changing our mindset can positively change our menopause experience at this natural stage of life. The simple yoga techniques give us tools that may change the way we physically feel. And the medical and wellbeing guidance can support our long-term health.

WHY THIS BOOK?

This is a practical yoga and wellbeing guide for busy people that gives you short daily practices. By making yoga accessible and achievable, I hope you will make it a daily habit and gain its therapeutic benefits.

The classes in this book can be used alongside other exercise and wellbeing programmes.

The practices are portable, so take them with you wherever you are: at home, staying in a hotel or during a break at work. Each class focuses on a specific symptom and includes bite-sized advice on wellbeing plus a Menopause Yoga short capsule class (5, 15, 30 minutes).

Each capsule class includes:

- Breathing techniques
- Accessible yoga poses
- A meditation/guided visualization/yoga nidra
- A journaling prompt
- A poem (where appropriate).

WHO IS THIS BOOK FOR?

Anyone can practise Menopause Yoga. It is designed to be accessible for people of all levels, from beginners to experienced yoga practitioners. It offers modifications to make the poses (asanas), breathing exercises (pranayama) and meditations suitable for your individual needs. The video classes aim to show a diversity of ethnicity, body shapes, ages and stages of the menopause.

A NOTE ON LANGUAGE

Cisgender women, non-binary people and transgender men all have a menopause if they have ovaries. This is because they are all affected by the fluctuations and decline of hormones in the ovaries. This change may destabilize the effects of their other hormone therapy and medications, causing unwanted symptoms and side effects.

To express inclusivity, I use both the words women and people in this book to reflect the diversity of lived experiences.

Not all people go through the menopause at midlife and not all are parents of children. I have tried to reflect this in the book.

You are unique.

Menopause is a unique experience for everyone. Many factors, like your genes, lifestyle choices and even your background, can influence how you go through it. Don't feel discouraged if your experience is different from others. The UK's National Institute for Health and Care Excellence (NICE) and the British Menopause Society (BMS) state that doctors should 'Adopt an individualized approach' to managing their patient's menopause[1] – and so should you. There is more information on diversity in Part One (see 'Diversity and difference: Why do I feel differently to others?').

HOW TO USE THIS BOOK

This book encourages you to create your own toolbox of self-care strategies and find what works best for *you*. Embrace your individuality and treat yourself with kindness and compassion.

I have included a variety of tools (poses, breathing exercises, meditations) and given alternative techniques for many of these in case you find them difficult. Don't worry about Sanskrit chants or acrobatic and pretzel poses. Focus on how each element makes you feel. If something feels uncomfortable (physically, mentally or emotionally), stop and do what feels safe for you. That particular yoga pose may not be right for you today, but try it again another time and it could be a gamechanger.

I have filmed short videos for you to watch to accompany the 'MY class' plans, and there are QR codes throughout the book for these. Alternatively, you can watch all the videos on my YouTube channel.* Explore the videos to find what works best for you. I have also included illustrated class sequences.

WHERE TO START

In 'Daily Practices', I have given some guidance to help you design your first home practice:

- A symptoms checklist to prioritize what you need today (see Part One). Remember, this will change over time as you move from perimenopause to menopause, then on to early postmenopause to Second Spring, and then Second Summer and beyond!
- A SMART goal template to decide what you want to gain from your practice, when, how often and why (see Part Three).

* www.youtube.com/@PetraMenopauseYoga

If you are not experiencing any specific symptoms, start by practising the suggested morning, afternoon or evening classes, and learn the stress-reducing skills in Part Four ('MY class to reduce stress').

Part One

WHAT IS THE MENOPAUSE?

History

The end of a woman's menstruation has been recorded throughout history, but it was the ancient Greek philosopher Aristotle, in 350 BC, who called it the 'climacteric', meaning a turning point in life. Modern medicine still uses the **Greene Climacteric Scale**[*] to assess if you are in the menopause.

The end of menstruation was observed to be the end of a woman's reproductivity, which many cultures viewed negatively. A woman's worth was measured by her ability to bear children (male heirs to property and wealth) and, without an understanding of female hormones and biology, the end of reproductivity was shrouded in fear and superstition. While some societies respected and revered older 'wise women', and valued their grandmother child-caring role, they also risked being seen as an economic burden, and in Western Europe lived in fear of being accused as witches and killed.

To this day, the social taboos around menopause, the misogyny surrounding the end of a woman's reproductivity, and the negative depiction of older (postmenopausal) women may subconsciously affect your view of menopause. Instead of seeing this as a positive natural time in your life to be embraced, you may feel an emotional resistance to 'The Change'.

Please do not blame yourself for these feelings; we all subconsciously absorb these attitudes that have been passed down through history in our culture, including through paintings, literature and songs depicting older women as frightening hags. Our grey hair, wrinkled skin and occasional facial hair is portrayed as ugly, at best, or we simply become invisible in public life. Menopause Yoga aims to change that negative narrative and

---

[*]   See, for example, https://appnhs24wp41a8c38o64.blob.core.windows.net/blobappn-hs24wp41a8c38o64/wp-content/uploads/2023/06/menopause-symptom-questionnaire_accessible-form-25_03_2022.pdf

reframe our menopause positively as our Second Spring, and to honour older women and people for their lived experiences and knowledge.

A MODERN MEDICAL PERSPECTIVE

The medical term 'la ménopause' was created by a French doctor, Charles Pierre Louis de Gardanne, in 1821, who combined the ancient Greek words *menos* (month) and *pauses* (end), and defined this as a sickness or syndrome needing treatment. This led to dangerous experimental surgery, toxic vaginal douches, injections of animal hormones and subsequent fatalities. The first hormone replacement therapy (HRT) was developed in the 1940s but fell out of fashion following health concerns. In the 1960s a newer version of oestrogen hormone therapy was promoted by Robert Wilson in his book *Feminine Forever*,[1] calling it the 'fountain of youth', and it was marketed to husbands for their wives. Later versions of HRT were deemed safer, until early results from the Women's Health Initiative research raised the alarm that HRT may increase the risk of breast cancer and other health risks.[2]

This research has now been discredited, and the International Menopause Society and doctors now recommend modern versions of HRT with lower health risks for a range of menopausal symptoms. However, there are still some risks you should be aware of, as well as myths and misinformation surrounding the menopause. So, in this next section, I invited Dr Claire Phipps, BSC MBBS MRCGP, a GP and Advanced Menopause Specialist and British Menopause Society (BMS) accredited trainer, to provide clear, factual information explaining the menopause, why it happens, medical definitions for the different stages, and modern hormone therapy options – for people who can, and want, to take it. Dr Phipps and the BMS state clearly that not everyone should, or needs to, take HRT. They also recommend lifestyle changes that may ease symptoms and reduce long-term health conditions after menopause.

Perimenopause and menopause*

Dr. Claire Phipps BSC MBBS MRCGP

WHAT IS PERIMENOPAUSE?

Perimenopause is the transition phase leading up to your last period. The menopause is caused by the natural decline in production of the hormones oestrogen and progesterone from your ovaries. This marks the end of a person's reproductive stage.

The ovaries (and the eggs within) produce oestrogen, which is one of the hormones that drives the natural reproductive cycle in women. As the number of eggs declines with age, so too does the production of oestrogen, and it is the fluctuation and decline in oestrogen that drives perimenopause symptoms.

WHAT AND WHEN IS MENOPAUSE?

Menopause is the medical term for one day in time when your periods have stopped for 12 consecutive months (in the absence of other health conditions). Before this you are perimenopausal and after, postmeno-pausal. The average age of menopause in the UK is 51, with most people experiencing menopause between the ages of 45 and 55 as a natural part of biological ageing.

Menopause that occurs between the ages of 40 and 45 is termed 'early menopause'. A spontaneous (natural) early menopause affects approximately 5 per cent of the population before the age of 45. It can be caused

---

* This section, up to 'Key takeaways', has been written by Dr Claire Phipps. See www. topdoctors.co.uk/doctor/claire-phipps

by treatment for other conditions such as surgery, chemotherapy or radiotherapy, for example.

HOW IS MENOPAUSE DIAGNOSED?

Women over the age of 45 who have any of the symptoms of perimenopause do not need any blood tests to diagnose menopause. This is because at this age and beyond it is highly likely that the natural decline in oestrogen has started to occur. Blood tests for hormone levels at this time are unreliable as they can fluctuate wildly. A normal result does not change the management of any symptoms if you are over the age of 45. However, your healthcare professional may opt to measure some bloods to ensure a holistic approach to your care.

Prior to the age of 45, and certainly in younger women, doctors may carry out some hormone blood tests and other blood profiles to rule menopause in or out. This is because in some people menopause can occur earlier, and it is important to clarify the cause, if possible, to provide the most appropriate treatment. It is important to rule out other causes of symptoms that can mimic menopausal symptoms too.

WHAT ARE COMMON SYMPTOMS OF PERIMENOPAUSE AND MENOPAUSE, WHY DO THEY HAPPEN AND CAN YOU TREAT THEM?

Symptoms and symptom severity will differ between people, and there may be times when symptoms are worse than at other times. You may also notice having a particular set of symptoms that then disappear completely. Again, this is due to the natural fluctuations in hormone levels occurring. Oestrogen is a master regulator of many processes in a woman's body, and as the levels decline or fluctuate, as they do (unpredictably), various physiological processes are affected, leading to physical, psychological and genitourinary symptoms.

Around 80 per cent of women will experience some degree of symptoms, and while some will not be severe, 25 per cent of women will have significant symptoms that might have a significant impact on their quality of life.

You may experience some of these symptoms at different times, or none.

Symptoms checklist

- Irregular periods. Menstrual cycles may become irregular in length and flow due to fluctuations in hormone levels, particularly oestrogen and progesterone. It is important to note, however, that periods can remain regular and you can still be perimenopausal.
- Hot flushes and night sweats. These sudden feelings of warmth, often accompanied by flushing of the face and upper body, can disrupt sleep and cause discomfort.
- Sleep disturbances. Changes in hormone levels can lead to insomnia, difficulty staying asleep or waking up frequently during the night.
- Vaginal dryness. Decreased oestrogen levels can result in vaginal dryness, itching and discomfort during intercourse, along with recurrent urine infections, burning and bleeding after intercourse. As levels of oestrogen fall, the vulval skin can become thinner, and it is common to need to pass urine more frequently.
- Mental health/psychological symptoms. Hormonal fluctuations can affect neurotransmitters in the brain, leading to mood swings, irritability, anxiety or depression.
- Changes in libido. Some women may experience a decrease in sexual desire or changes in sexual function during perimenopause.
- Fatigue. Hormonal changes, disrupted sleep and other symptoms can contribute to feelings of tiredness and fatigue.
- Weight gain. Changes in hormone levels and metabolism can make it easier to gain weight, especially around the abdomen. Weight gain, however, is not inevitable.
- Memory problems and difficulty concentrating. Some women may experience cognitive changes such as forgetfulness, difficulty concentrating or 'brain fog'.
- Muscle and joint pains.
- Dry eyes and dry skin.

TREATMENT FOR SYMPTOMS

An individualized approach is necessary in managing symptoms of menopause, with a variety of treatment choices available. Treatment options usually depend on the severity of your symptoms, type of symptoms and your personal preferences, and should always take into consideration your medical and family history.

Options include hormone replacement therapy (HRT), which aims to supplement and stabilize the hormones that the ovaries were producing so that the symptoms and effects of menopause are minimized.

Hormone replacement therapy

The two main hormones in HRT are oestrogen and a progestogen. HRT involves either taking both of these hormones (combined HRT) or, in the case of women who have had a total hysterectomy, taking oestrogen alone (oestrogen-only HRT). Oestrogen causes the lining of the womb to thicken and progesterone stops the lining from getting too thick.

There are some people who, following a hysterectomy, still take progestogen. This is part of an individualized discussion with your healthcare provider. For example, women who have had severe endometriosis may be advised to use progestogen alongside oestrogen.

HRT should always be started after a careful assessment of risks and benefits and after a full discussion about all treatment options so that you can make an informed decision. It is all about choice.

Today, we aim to use body identical preparations. Essentially this means hormones that are identical to what our ovaries produced. We aim to use oestrogen that is delivered through the skin (also known as transdermal oestrogen). Taking oestrogen through the skin does not increase the risk of blood clots or strokes, and it can be taken as a patch, spray or gel.

'Body identical progesterone' refers to the progesterone that is chemically identical to the hormone produced naturally in the body. There are a few different products available depending on the country you live in. It is taken as an oral capsule at night as it can have soporific effects – which, for many women for whom sleep is a problem, can be helpful.

If you are still having your periods, body identical progesterone is taken for part of the month. If you are no longer having periods, it is taken every night. If you have a womb, it is important that you are using progestogen to protect the lining of the womb from becoming too thick.

There are many different progestogen options available in addition to body identical progesterone. It may take time to find the right combination of HRT (both oestrogen and progestogen) for you, and the dose of progestogen needs to be adequate for the amount of oestrogen that you are using. The decision on which type of progestogen to take will depend on many different things, and needs to be individualized and discussed carefully. HRT can also be taken in tablet form.

Contraception

It is worth remembering that you are still fertile in the perimenopause, so contraception still needs to be considered. The Mirena coil can be a good contraceptive choice and also doubles as the progestogenic component of your HRT for up to five years. Progesterone-only contraception can also be used and can be taken safely alongside HRT.

Genitourinary syndrome of menopause

'Genitourinary syndrome of menopause' (GSM) refers to the collection of symptoms and physical changes that affect the genital and urinary systems during the perimenopause and beyond due to the decline in oestrogen.

Around 80 per cent of women will experience some degree of GSM symptoms. The vaginal lining becomes dryer and much more delicate. This can lead to discomfort during sex, bleeding after sex, recurrent urine infections, thrush, generalized discomfort, burning, itching and bladder weakness.

These symptoms respond well to topical vaginal oestrogen treatment. This is not HRT and can be used safely alongside HRT or on its own. If you only use topical vaginal oestrogen treatment, you do not need to use a progestogen. Depending on your symptoms and their severity, topical vaginal oestrogen can be used as a cream, gel or pessary, or a flexible ring inserted into the vagina.

Lack of libido can be a common symptom in the perimenopause and postmenopause as our ovaries produce less testosterone, which can reduce sexual desire. HRT can often help, but, if severe, seeing your doctor is important as treatment requires a whole person approach.

ALTERNATIVES TO HRT AND LIFESTYLE OPTIONS

If you choose not to use HRT, or cannot use HRT for medical reasons, there are many prescribable alternatives.

Regardless of whether you take HRT or not, a holistic approach is key – lifestyle, nutrition, cognitive behavioural therapy (CBT), acupuncture, exercise and mindful movement, including yoga, are fundamental in helping to manage symptoms.

KEY TAKEAWAYS

- Menopause is a natural phase in a woman's life, typically occurring between the ages of 45 and 55, marking the end of menstruation and reproductive ability due to declining hormone levels.

- Treatment options focus on alleviating these symptoms and main-taining overall health. Hormone replacement therapy (HRT) can help stabilize your hormone levels, while non-hormonal medi-cations can help those who cannot take HRT or who choose not to take it. Lifestyle changes, such as a healthy diet, regular exer-cise, mindful movement such as yoga and stress management, are crucial.

- Overarching all of this is the importance of discussing any of your symptoms with your doctor so that you can be supported holistically.

Your Symptoms

The figure on the following page shows many of the symptoms associated with menopause – tick the ones that you are experiencing.

Which symptoms do you have that are missing from the figure? There are 34 recognized symptoms of menopause, including: tinnitus, vertigo, fear of driving, dry eyes and mouth, hair thinning and loss, gum disease and dental issues – and more! You may experience different symptoms at different stages of perimenopause to postmenopause – or none at all. Some people experience severe symptoms but for others these are mild.

Headache

Systemic
- Weight gain
- Heavy night sweats

Palpitations

Breasts
- Enlargement
- Pain

Skin
- Hot flashes
- Dryness
- Itching
- Thinning
- Tingling

Joints
- Soreness
- Stiffness

Back pain

Urinary
- Incontinence
- Urgency

Psychological
- Dizziness
- Interrupted
  sleeping patterns
- Anxiety
- Poor memory
- Inability to
  concentrate
- Depressive mood
- Irritability
- Mood swings
- Less interest in
  sexual activity

Transitional
menstruations
- Shorter or
  longer cycles
- Bleeding between
  periods

Vaginal
- Dryness
- Painful
  intercourse

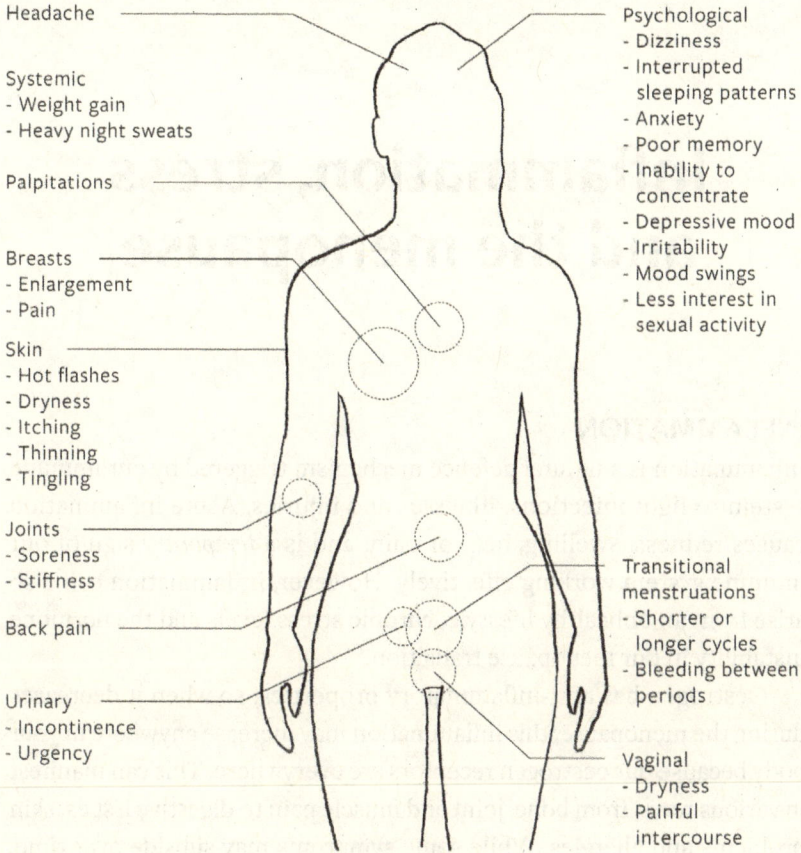

SYMPTOMS BODY

IS MENOPAUSE GETTING WORSE?

Modern life is affecting menopause. We are leading more sedentary lives, exercising less, eating unhealthy ultra-processed foods and working indoors for longer hours, and many of us consume caffeine stimulants in the day and alcohol relaxants in the evenings to wind down. Social isolation, discrimination and financial instability may also contribute to increased stress levels, which may make our symptoms worse and impact our long-term health.

Inflammation, stress and the menopause

INFLAMMATION

Inflammation is a natural defence mechanism triggered by our immune system to fight infections, illnesses and injuries. Acute inflammation causes redness, swelling, heat or pain, and is a *temporary* sign of our immune system working effectively. However, inflammation can also arise from an unhealthy lifestyle, chronic stress levels and the hormone instability in our menopause transition.[3]

Oestrogen has anti-inflammatory properties, so when it decreases during the menopause, this inflammation may increase anywhere in your body because our oestrogen receptors are everywhere. This can manifest in various ways, from bone, joint and muscle pain to digestive issues, skin problems and allergies. While some symptoms may subside over time, chronic inflammation in postmenopausal women increases long-term health risks.

Chronic stress isn't an anomaly; nowadays it's the norm. The boundaries of work and home have become blurred, making us constantly available and less able to switch off our digital devices – or our brains. The stress we bring with us as we enter perimenopause will affect our physical, psychological and emotional symptoms – and health risks. Menopause is a wake-up call!

STRESS FACTORS

Are you feeling overloaded? The average woman goes through menopause at midlife, which is when a confluence of life circumstances may converge, causing stress, and include: bereavement, divorce, redundancy or changes at work, and children reaching adolescence or leaving home. Managing these stress factors may have been easy in the past but, in the menopause, your brain may struggle to cope. If you have children later in life, your postnatal drop in hormones may push you straight into perimenopause. If you feel unable to cope with stress, this is called allostatic overload.[4]

Hormone see-saw

High levels of chronic (long-term) stress in your nervous system affect your endocrine system. Similar to a see-saw, the higher your levels of stress chemicals, cortisol and adrenaline, the lower your levels of oestrogen, progesterone and testosterone (OPT). Racial, ethnic, gender identity and religious discrimination are factors that may lead to attritional stress. This is believed to be one of the reasons why people from these discriminated groups may enter menopause earlier – because their endocrine system is overloaded by lifetime attritional stress (see 'Diversity and difference: Why do I feel differently to others?').

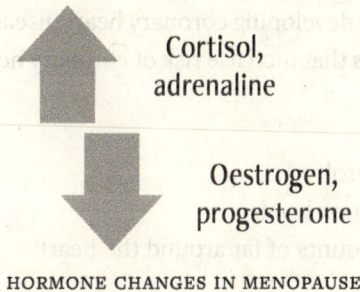

Cortisol,
adrenaline

Oestrogen,
progesterone

HORMONE CHANGES IN MENOPAUSE

Long-term health risks

After menopause, there are increased health risks that are partly due to ageing, but some particularly affect women. These include cardiovascular disease, osteoporosis, cancer, type 2 diabetes, dementia and depression.

Heart

Coronary heart disease is a major cause of death for women over the age of 50, and oestrogen has a protective effect on the heart. When oestrogen levels fall, fat can accumulate in arteries, causing narrowing and increasing the risk of developing coronary heart disease, a heart attack or stroke.[5] Body changes that increase risk of coronary heart disease include:

- Weight gain
- High cholesterol
- High blood sugar levels
- Increased amounts of fat around the heart.

Bones

Osteoporosis is a condition that weakens bones and increases fracture risk. This can occur after menopause as female hormones (oestrogen, progesterone and testosterone) support the renewal of skeletal material.

Women experience a more rapid decline in bone density during the first five years of menopause, losing up to 10 per cent of their bone mass. Smaller bone size can increase the risk of osteoporosis, along with genetics, low body weight, unhealthy diet and over-exercising.[6]

Breasts

Breast cancer is the most common cancer affecting women in the UK, and the risk increases after menopause, with around 80 per cent of breast cancers diagnosed in women over 50. The postmenopausal risk is due to ageing in combination with hormonal changes affecting cell growth. Early detection through screening means that eight out of ten women diagnosed with breast cancer at this stage survive.[7]

Diabetes and weight gain

Up to 70 per cent of women experience body composition changes during menopause and postmenopause. Fat (adipose) storage shifts from the hips and thighs (pear-shaped) to the abdomen (apple-shaped), affecting around 50 per cent of postmenopausal women. This shift, linked to declining oestrogen, can lead to insulin resistance, a condition affecting up to 30 per cent of postmenopausal women, and even those with a healthy weight.[8]

Muscles

Weaker muscle tissue (sarcopenia or atrophy) is one of the most important causes of functional decline and loss of independence as we get older. Potential causes include the menopause decline in hormone levels as well as physical activity, insufficient protein in the diet, poor sleep and increased oxidative stress.[9]

Brain

Dementia is a decline in cognitive abilities impacting daily life, and while ageing is the main cause of dementia, an estimated 65 per cent of people affected are women.[10]

Mental health

Oestrogen and progesterone help regulate the brain's levels of serotonin, dopamine, noradrenaline and oxytocin, which make us feel happy, grounded and connected to others. While some people will have a history of clinical depression, others may experience mental health issues for the first time in their menopause.

Menopause psychological symptoms include low mood or anhedonia (where you feel flat, like a grey cloud is hanging over your head), generalized anxiety, feeling overwhelmed, mood swings such as irritability or tearfulness, migraine headaches, low self-confidence, social withdrawal and sleep disturbance. Cognitive symptoms include brain fog and difficulties with memory retrieval or concentration. The good news is that these symptoms do not last forever. Neuroscientist Dr Lisa Mosconi says brain symptoms are not necessarily long term, because cognitive function 'bounces back' in postmenopause if we reduce stress and lead a healthy lifestyle.[11]

There is so much you can do for yourself, such as eating a healthy (Mediterranean) diet, regular exercise and restful sleep (see Part Two: Health and Wellbeing). Stress management is crucial for everyone going through the menopause to ameliorate the impact on the endocrine (hormone) system. Yoga is proven to help reduce stress reduction (see 'MY class to reduce stress', and 'Beyond yoga: Techniques for menopause stress reduction'. Skip forward to Part Three: Yoga Basics and Part Four: Daily Practices if you want to dive into the yoga practice.

Diversity and difference: Why do I feel differently to others?

Do you feel like your friends are breezing through their menopause while you are still struggling with symptoms? Maybe you have started menopause earlier than others, or wonder why the latest wonder 'cure' everyone raves about didn't help you?

Please be reassured, this is normal because your experience of your menopause is uniquely individual. The National Institute for Health and Care Excellence (NICE) advises doctors in the UK to 'adopt an individualised approach at all stages of diagnosis, investigation and management of perimenopause and menopause'.[12]

These different experiences may be due to your genetics, or how sensitive you are to hormone change, lifestyle and lived experience. Lived experience may be entering menopause earlier than average due to premature ovarian insufficiency (POI), mothering small children in perimenopause, medically induced menopause, or emotional trauma, including discrimination due to ethnicity and gender identity.

You may once have chosen to not have children, but now feel the choice is no longer yours to make. You may be grieving elderly parents or your own loss of identity. Here, I have invited experts to share their insights into diversity of experience in the menopause. If their stories resonate with you, please remember that you are not alone (see the Resources section at the end of this book for help and information).

PREMATURE OVARIAN INSUFFICIENCY

POI is a condition where the ovaries do not function as they should and occurs before the age of 40. Unlike early menopause, people with POI may still have occasional periods, and approximately 4–10 per cent of those diagnosed may go on to conceive naturally. Commonly, women have irregular or no periods for four to six months or more, and have symptoms consistent with perimenopause.[13]

Causes of POI range from autoimmune diseases, genetic conditions, some infection, and sometimes, no cause is found. A diagnosis of early menopause or POI requires an integrated approach from a wide range of healthcare professionals to provide individualized support.[14]

MY POI STORY

Who would have thought the menopause would come early for me? Nobody warned me, nobody in the family went through it that way. But here I was, age 32, without a period for months and with a whole lot of uncomfortable symptoms. I had premature ovarian insufficiency (POI), also known as premature menopause. There was a lot of grief, for the genetic child I would probably never have, for my loss of identity as a young, fertile woman, and for that future family I had always imagined. I was also scared about ageing. What happens to your body when you become infertile? Are you catapulted into the body of an old woman from one day to the next? Nobody talks about this. It is all such a taboo...to the point that I didn't even know it would be possible to go into menopause at this early age!

The first years dealing with my POI diagnosis were extremely difficult, filled with insecurities, questions and loneliness; however, HRT, yoga and surrounding myself with a community of supportive women helped me greatly.

(For support and information, visit the Daisy Network.*)

Veronica Santini, yoga teacher, somatic coach and founder of Tales of Her

TRAUMA

According to the World Health Organization (WHO), 70 per cent of people will experience at least one significant traumatic event in their

---

*   www.daisynetwork.org

lifetime.[15] These traumatic experiences impact our physical health. Hala Khouri, yoga teacher and psychologist, explains: 'Traumatic events are events that overwhelm our capacity to cope and respond, leaving us feeling helpless, hopeless, and out of control. Events themselves are not inherently traumatic; it is our response that determines if the event was traumatic.'[16] Khouri goes on to explain that not all traumas come from major events (such as war, violent abuse or injury due to a car accident); some may be '"little t" everyday traumas'.[17] When we don't have the tools and resources to deal with traumatic events, they may impact our physical wellbeing and our mental health.

Caroline Phipps explains how this can directly impact menopause symptoms.

> Adrenaline and cortisol, the stress hormones, are designed to keep us safe from danger and ensure we have the energy to cope with the impending threat. These stress hormones increase due to anxiety, high-sugar foods including alcohol, and juggling busy lives; they also inhibit oestrogen and progesterone production. As our sex hormones fluctuate through perimenopause, this too can also trigger our stress response. If we have experienced trauma in our lived experience then our bodies know the stress path well, so it is imperative to have the tools to help support us through what can be a challenging time.
>
> Research shows that 'the experience of childhood abuse and neglect is associated with increased vasomotor symptom reporting in adulthood', leading to more severe vasomotor symptoms (e.g., hot flushes) in midlife, particularly through menopause.[18] Further research suggests that a lifetime history of intimate partner violence (IPV) or sexual assault leads to a 50 per cent higher chance of suffering from night sweats and 60 per cent higher odds of painful sex.[19] These women demonstrate clinically significant symptoms of posttraumatic stress disorder (PTSD) associated with menopause symptoms, and this highlights the need for greater awareness by clinicians caring for midlife and older women. Talking therapies obviously can help, and we also know that breathing and somatic movement, like yoga, can encourage the release of these emotions that get stuck in the body.
>
> *Caroline Phipps, trauma-informed breathwork & yoga therapist*

My therapist used to say the trauma I had experienced through childhood was like a rock in the pit of my stomach. I had grown around it; it had remained deep inside me, rooted, buried. Its heaviness weighed me down for what felt like an eternity, then through my work with my therapist it became lighter. I now describe my rock as having soft edges. Historically, the connections I made with others were always determined by my lived experience in the family home. I was on high alert, looking for red flags or otherwise people-pleasing by rarely vocalizing my wants and needs. The foundation of my relationships steeped in my mother's temper. I can now, with distance, recognize my mother's temper as hormonal; the stress response activated around my mother's monthly cycle exacerbated by her menopause and most likely also a consequence of her own trauma experience. As I navigate perimenopause I find I am increasingly grateful to have my yoga practice to support me. From menorage to low mood, the years of practice have given me a toolkit to draw upon to alleviate symptoms – breathwork, yoga nidra, asana and meditation.

Charlotte Lowther

ETHNICITY

When I ask my mum about her menopause, she either doesn't remember, or doesn't want to talk about it. Some of this is generational: when I ask my 50-something white or Asian friends about their mums, it's often the same. Some is cultural: I'm West Indian and we don't really talk about that stuff.

It doesn't help that the conversation around menopause hasn't often included black voices. When you grow up in a country where you're seen as 'other' it's normal for your voice to not be counted. But this doesn't make it okay.

Well-documented health disparities can't help but feed into black women's mistrust of the health profession. When you hear that black women are five times more likely to die in childbirth than their white counterparts, or that fibroids are the cause of 30 per cent of hysterectomies in white women, but 50 per cent of hysterectomies in black women, you can perhaps understand why.

Patsy Isles, a writer, media skills trainer and yoga teacher

---

*   See www.patsyisles.com and www.ifeyoga.com

A person's ethnicity can affect their experience of menopause in numerous ways. In the UK, approximately 13 per cent of the population are from Black, Asian, mixed or other ethnic groups. The overall impact on physical symptoms of menopause shows there are health inequalities that women of colour face disproportionately. These span from low levels of awareness to evidence of failure to provide treatment by medical practitioners. A Fawcett Society survey of 4000 people in the UK found that 45 per cent of women of colour said it took many appointments before their GP diagnosed menopause as the cause of their symptoms.[20]

Dr Radhika Vohra, an NHS doctor in the UK with a special interest in women's health and menopause, says women from lower socioeconomic groups are 30 per cent less likely to be prescribed HRT than those from more affluent areas, with symptoms that are often misdiagnosed, and higher levels of chronic and metabolic diseases. Dr Vohra says:

Women of colour are more likely to experience long-lasting chronic stress and this can cause 'allostatic overload'. 'Allostatic load' refers to the strain on the body and when excessive, the body goes into 'overload' and presents with symptoms such as sleep disturbances, irritability, impaired social or occupational functioning, and feelings of being overwhelmed by the demands of daily life. If it persists, allostatic overload affects hormonal balance and may ultimately result in physical and/or mental health problems.[21]

Research also shows that women of colour have higher rates of obesity, dyslipidaemia, hypertension and impaired glucose metabolism, and increased risk of cardiovascular disease. Genetics-based differences in insulin sensitivity and body mass index were also reported.[22]

If you identify as a person of colour, please seek advice from your doctor or a medical professional who you feel comfortable talking with. See also organizations listed in the Resources section at the end of the book.

From my own experience, the systemic racism in our society means the voice of other black and brown women were lost or not wanted. It took longer to acknowledge our own debilitating symptoms and begin to care for ourselves. We are finally finding allies within the wellness communities who champion our voices and respectfully move aside for our voices to be heard. I am grateful that today I see many black and brown faces sharing their menopause experiences and writing their stories. I see myself in books and research – I share spaces with women of all colours, and we are starting to see each other and welcome our differences and speak our truths together. This is what gives me hope that with small societal change, we will one day be on the same playing field with much better outcomes for all who experience life-changing menopause symptoms.[23]

Ayana Williams, a yoga teacher and founder of Movement for the Menopause

TREATMENT-INDUCED MENOPAUSE

Endometriosis treatment may include surgery to remove the ovaries, or an induced menopause by supressing a person's menstrual cycle to reduce the level of oestrogen produced by their ovaries.[24]

If you have undergone surgical menopause (a hysterectomy or oophorectomy), the onset of your menopause symptoms may be sudden and more severe due to the immediate loss of hormones produced in your ovaries.

Vasomotor symptoms such as hot flushes, joint and muscle pain, loss of libido, anxiety and mood changes and urogenital symptoms (vaginal dryness and urinary tract infections) are common side effects, and you may be at higher risk of cardiovascular disease and osteoporosis. HRT plays a significant role in managing surgical menopause, especially in women under the age of 45 (provided there are no contraindications such as a personal history or hormone-dependent cancer). Non-pharmacological options include exercise, weight management and cognitive behavioural therapy (CBT). Your emotional wellbeing may also be affected by the immediate end of your reproductivity as a result of this surgery, so your doctor should offer you professional counselling.[25]

CANCER IN MENOPAUSE

Globally, 9 million women are diagnosed with cancer each year, and breast cancer is the most commonly diagnosed cancer worldwide. While survival from cancer is improving, the medical treatment can trigger premature ovarian insufficiency (POI) or early menopause. Managing menopausal symptoms after cancer can be more severe than at natural menopause, and challenging to manage.

Treatment-induced symptoms can include hot flushes and night sweats as well as genitourinary issues, and impaired sleep, mood and quality of life. Recent research published in *The Lancet* medical journal suggests that HRT 'is an effective treatment for vasomotor symptoms and seems to be safe for many patients with cancer'. And further, 'Vaginal oestrogen seems safe for most patients with genitourinary symptoms.'[26] However, many women are advised by their doctor or choose not to take HRT.[27]

For people with oestrogen receptor cancer, there are also potential risks associated with non-hormonal treatments, such as nutrition and herbal remedies if they contain natural phytoestrogen that mimics oestrogen in the body.

Yoga can benefit people before, during and after cancer treatment and surgery (see 'MY class for breast cancer recovery').

NEURODIVERSITY: AUTISM AND ADHD IN WOMEN

WHAT IT'S LIKE HAVING AUTISM IN MENOPAUSE

My heightened senses in perimenopause has made it almost impossible for me to function as I was. The world had become too overwhelming, the noise, the smells, the bright lighting, everyday tasks and peopleing. The masking and scripting I have done most of my life serve me no more; I did not have the energy, which led to meltdowns and shutdowns, my nervous system in flight, fight or, more commonly for me, freeze or fawn. Unmasking has not been an easy process, but it brings so much more confidence and fulfilment.

Jinty Sheerin, podcaster, co-host of WomenKind Collective podcast

The characteristics of autism and ADHD in women may be different to autistic men and boys, possibly because women 'mask' their traits more effectively. However, the stress of constantly masking to 'fit in' can result in anxiety and overwhelm. Research into women with neurodiversity is limited (at the time of writing), but emerging experts in this field, such as Adele Wimsett, are observing how women with neurodiversity appear to unravel in their perimenopause, possibly due to the hormonal rewiring of the brain and the higher levels of stress experienced causing allostatic overload.[28]

Women's health practitioner with a specialist interest in ADHD, Adele Wimsett, says many women go undiagnosed until later life.

ADHD AND PERIMENOPAUSE

As women get closer towards menopause hormone changes, it can feel like you're dropping off a cliff because the ADHD traits become more severe. The lid feels like it has literally come off. You might think 'I'm scared. I feel like I'm going crazy. What's happening to me? Nothing's working. I used to cope so well. I was superwomen. I did all these things and now I just can't do it.' This is because the support we've usually have for our neurotransmitters from the oestrogen and progesterone is no longer there. At certain times in the menstrual cycle when oestrogen withdraws, traits go through the roof and we may switch between inattentiveness and hyperactivity.

Women with ADHD may experience a challenging menopause, and this is really important as many have spent their lives silencing their experience because they've been told they're too dramatic. For most women, proges-terone sensitizes something called gamma-aminobutyric acid (GABA) in the brain, which is a neurotransmitter that produces a calming, relaxing, sleep-inducing effect. Symptoms associated with deficiencies are reported in your early 40s when feelings of anxiety, being overwhelmed and sleep disruption occur. We need to find strategies that calm us and work for us. Yoga can help by calming and regulating our nervous system, so that cortisol, insulin and inflammation decrease.

*Adele Wimsett, from Harmonise You**

---

* See https://harmoniseyou.co.uk **and also** www.autism.org.uk/advice-and-guidance/topics/physical-health/menopause#Autism%20and%20the%20menopause

Gender identity and menopause

Until recently, research into queer and gender-diverse experiences of menopause has been limited. What is known is that assigned-female-at-birth, non-binary people and trans men all have a menopause experience, and the symptoms may be more challenging or be a psychological struggle. Trans men may take HRT to increase testosterone, but if their ovaries are still present, the fluctuations of OPT hormones can be psychologically and emotionally destabilizing. People who have ovaries but do not identify as a cisgender female may find the hormonal fluctuations force them back to a gender with which they do not identify.

Tania Glyde, a psychotherapist/counsellor specializing in gender, sex and relationships in diverse clients, says the discrimination that queer people face in the UK, and subsequent chronic stress, also contributes to the psychological symptoms in perimenopause. Research shows that trans and non-binary people are more vulnerable to mental health issues, and may have had a negative experience of medical treatment by mainstream doctors in the past.[29]

Dr Stella Duffy's research was on the embodied experience of postmenopause.

QUEERING MENOPAUSE

I became menopausal in my 30s, when chemotherapy for my first breast cancer pushed me into menopause, causing infertility just at the point my wife and I were trying for children. In my mid-50s, having been postmenopausal for decades, I embarked on a doctorate in existential psychotherapy. I chose to research *post*menopause,[30] not least to combat the disturbingly prevalent idea that menopause is the end, rather than a transition to a new phase of life. I offer below some possibilities for more generous inclusion of LGBTQIA+ experience.

Why it's different for us

Our society is predicated on the idea that everyone is heterosexual, heterosexuality is the norm, and the gender binary is true for all. For those of us for whom this is not the case, there is a constant requirement to take what is offered and translate it to our own experience. This is both exhausting and relentless, as evidenced in Silas' research into the experience of everyday coming out, which eloquently attests to the emotional labour involved. Glyde has researched and written extensively about queer menopause,[31] but it remains the case that LGBTQIA+ menopausal experience has been largely disregarded by anyone other than queer researchers.

Why it's useful to include us

A great deal of the wider research suggests that some of what is problematic in menopause is a sense of becoming invisible in older age.[32] Queer people have often had to either be invisible, in order to protect ourselves from antagonism and abuse, or been made invisible by a culture that denies our existence. Our lived experience of this imposition can therefore be useful for our heterosexual siblings as we all experience a further layer of being made invisible as we age in an ageist culture.

Body image

Body changes in menopause are conventionally described as problematic, especially around weight gain and shape change, when the body shifts from that which is usually deemed of value in white heteronormative culture – the slender, conventionally attractive body presenting a youthful image of fertility (with fertility assumed to equal value) – to an ageing body with different weight distribution that likely does not conform to the standard sociocultural depictions of attractiveness.

The possibility that we might appreciate our bodies, regardless of how they fit into the dictates of heteronormative society and fashion, offers me hope that ageing might free us from some of the constraints imposed upon most of us since our teens.

Sexual intimacy in menopause and beyond

The vast majority of representations of sexual intimacy throughout white Western culture are of heterosexuality with a standard implication that penis-in-vagina sex is the only sex that actually matters. Non-heterosexual intimacy, however, opens possibilities for more consideration of what partners actually want from sex and what they might be open to explore as their bodies change over time. While people in any relationship can engage in these vital intimate conversations, being outside the heteronorm makes the discussion of what we *actually* desire rather more likely. Interviews with lesbian and heterosexual women about the impact of menopause on their sex lives, found that:

> None of the lesbians describe partners who complain about menopause, and many accounts illustrate female sexual agency because women openly discuss sex and act on their desires.[33]

*Dr Stella Duffy, a psychotherapist, writer and yoga teacher**

---

* See https://stelladuffytherapy.co.uk

Reframing menopause: From symptoms to Second Spring

A POSITIVE MINDSET

Menopause has had a negative press; it needs a rebrand. Instead of viewing this stage of life as a list of symptoms, and our years ahead as being filled with doom and gloom, we can own our menopause and reframe it positively. There is so much more to your menopause. It is an awakening to your self and a wake-up call to change what is no longer nourishing and supporting you. Your B.S. filter lifts and you may suddenly feel the urge to call out injustice and unfairness in society, and feel outraged. This means you become a positive force for change. You start stepping into your place of self-empowerment and leadership. You may feel a passion to start a new project, a surge of creativity or a desire to share your knowledge educationally with others. You're unstoppable – go for it!

And it's not just society that benefits from your new-found clarity and voice. Viewing your menopause positively may reduce your own levels of stress, which may ease some of your symptoms. Reframe your menopause as an opportunity for improving your health and happiness, allowing you to let go of past trauma, baggage that you don't want to take with you into the next stage of life.

I encourage you to embrace modern science and the wisdom of Eastern traditions to view your menopause as a dress rehearsal, or rite of passage, preparing you to step into your Second Spring.

Look forward to the menopause as:

- A positive pause. A chance for radical rest, self-compassion and acceptance.

- A wake-up call. An alarm bell to prioritize health and happiness, especially if chronic stress is present.
- A time to reflect and release. Empower yourself by choosing to let go of any habits, behaviours, negative thought patterns and the emotional pain attached to past memories. This will lighten your load and free you for the next stage in life.
- An awakening. A chance to rediscover creativity, confidence and zest for life in your Second Spring.

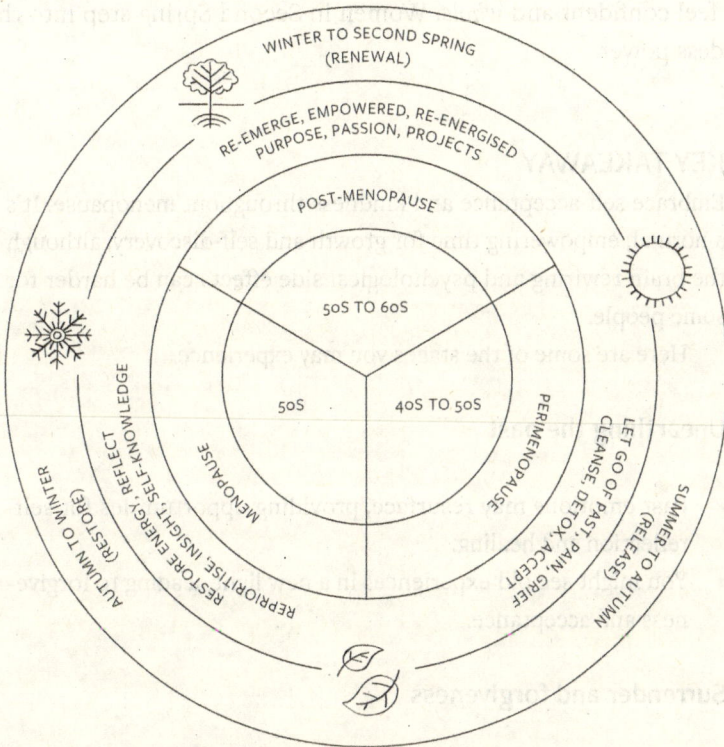

MENOPAUSE AGES, STAGES AND SEASONS

WHAT IS SECOND SPRING?

Second Spring is a time of new growth, a new lease of life in our post-menopausal years. Free from the cycle of ovulation and menstruation, our hormones become more stable in postmenopause, although it may take three to seven years to find a new equilibrium.[34]

According to Traditional Chinese Medicine (TCM), our Second Spring is when we are able to harness the energy we used to expend on the menstrual cycle and redirect it to new creative ventures and projects, or realize dreams that we did not have time for previously. It is an opportunity for self-fulfilment – to realize our potential. At this stage of life, there is an insight into our selves that feels empowering, an acceptance of who we are, with affection and understanding rather than judgement. This can be a liberating time of 'not caring what other people think', as we seek to please ourselves rather than others. This is a time when we can feel confident and *whole*. Women in Second Spring step into their goddess power.

KEY TAKEAWAY

Embrace self-acceptance and kindness throughout menopause. It's a normal, empowering time for growth and self-discovery, although the brain rewiring and psychological side effects can be harder for some people.

Here are some of the stages you may experience.

Unearthing the past

- Past emotions may resurface, providing opportunities for self-reflection and healing.
- You might see old experiences in a new light, leading to forgiveness and acceptance.

Surrender and forgiveness

- Letting go of past hurts and anger can be liberating.
- Forgive yourself and others in order to move forward without the burden of resentment.

Embracing yourself

- Every woman's experience is unique.
- Accept and embrace who you are, even the parts that feel embarrassing.

- Seek professional support if needed.

Normalizing mood swings

- Mood swings, fatigue and anger are common during menopause.
- Forgive yourself for unintentionally hurting others during these episodes.
- Expressing emotions is healthy.

Finding support

- If you are struggling, you don't need to do this on your own. Please seek professional counselling support (see the Resources section at the end of this book).

After Second Spring

Menopause is more than a medical term and a list of negative symptoms; it's a physical spring clean and a brain upgrade preparing you for a great awakening.

Petra Coveney

Your brain bounces back. Neuroscientist Dr Mosconi says the menopause cognitive symptoms, such as brain fog, memory retrieval and overwhelm, are part of a brain 'upgrade'.

In women's brain scans, Dr Mosconi observed that some brain function deemed unnecessary in postmenopause decreases (such as the breastfeeding response), but this is a natural positive spring clean designed to make your brain 'leaner and meaner, discarding information and skills it no longer needs while growing new ones... Once the update is complete, the symptoms start dissipating.'[35]

Dr Mosconi's research reveals that we have a postmenopause 'superpower', *empathy*, which is believed to be preparation for our next important societal role in later life:

So, it is not a weakness – it is our strength. We just didn't realise this because society told us we were less than or inferior without our fertility. It looks like society was wrong – and women are waking up to this. Let's look after our long-term health and get 'leaner and meaner'.[36]

In our 'Great Awakening' we may also lose our filter and find ourselves calling out unfairness, inequality and injustice. This new assertiveness and not giving a **** is also our superpower.

What did your teenage-self dream about? Carpe diem dear friends – what are you waiting for?

I've spoken to people in postmenopause who've embraced their teenage dreams and revved up their old motorbike to ride around India, rented a horse to go bareback riding, written a book of poems that was self-published to great acclaim, started a menopause campaign and won awards, begun a new health-related business, joined a choir and performed at a famous opera festival, or they started tap dancing, swimming or running marathons.

I hope some of you will find your voice and gain the self-confidence to turn your menopause rage into outrage to create social change. Do you feel ready to become the leaders of communities, business, politicians and environmental organizations, and help us protect this beautiful planet for future generations?

If that just sounds exhausting, then find pleasure after menopause and enjoy yourself. Do whatever makes you happy.

Listen to this Guided visualisation for Second Spring.

Part Two

HEALTH AND WELLBEING

Lifestyle changes can make a difference to your menopause symptoms and long-term health. Whether you are in perimenopause or postmenopause, it is never too early or too late to make simple changes to your daily life.

In this section, I have invited some of the most respected menopause experts to give you general guidance on nutrition, herbal remedies, Ayurveda, exercise, Nature and cold water swimming, cognitive behavioural therapy (CBT) and journaling.

This is a daily practice guide, aimed at making simple changes sustainable, so I suggest that you start with making *one* change to your nutrition, such as reducing alcohol, or coffee, or sugar. In the words of the late Dr Michael Mosley, for sustainable shifts in your lifestyle, change 'just *one* thing', not everything at once.[1]

I recommend that you keep a journal by your bed to note down if this makes a difference to your symptoms. Stick to this *one* change for *one* week (don't try everything at once) because you need to know if and how a substance affects you. You are a unique individual. For instance, do you notice less bloating, or fewer night sweats, or less anxiety?

When you have worked your way through reducing the foods and drinks that commonly disrupt our hormones in menopause, consider adding in the healthy nutritious suggestions made by Emma Ellice Flint in the following chapter. Then you may want to look at your levels of movement etc. This takes time, so be patient with yourself. It can be a wonderful journey of self-discovery, and an opportunity to press pause and reset your body, mind and emotions. What we needed in our 20s and 30s will be different from what nourishes us in our 40s and 50s. Enjoy the journey.

Nutrition

Emma Ellice Flint, nutritionist

Hormonal changes, particularly a decline in oestrogen, can trigger inflammation in the body. This inflammation, coupled with the associated stress, can lead to a range of symptoms that affect your wellbeing. These hormonal shifts can disrupt the balance of your gut microbiome, exacerbating inflammation such as mood changes. Here, nutritionist Emma Ellice Flint gives her advice on how you can reduce inflammation, and support your gut, health and wellbeing with what you eat and drink.

UNDERSTANDING THE CONNECTION BETWEEN INFLAMMATION AND SYMPTOMS

The increase in inflammation during perimenopause and menopause can manifest in various ways, including mood swings, irritability, headaches, mental fog, low energy, disrupted sleep and changes in skin, hair and nail quality. It can also lead to digestive issues like constipation, or loose bowel movements and gut bloating, as well as disruptions in blood sugar balance and potential weight gain. However, it's important to note that while these symptoms can be linked to hormonal changes and inflammation, they can also be caused by underlying medical conditions. Consult your doctor before making any dietary changes.

Balancing inflammation through food

Fortunately, you can take steps to manage and reduce inflammation through your food choices. Here are six fundamental dietary principles that have proven effective in supporting women during perimenopause and postmenopause:

1. Fibre and prebiotic foods

Fibre is often an overlooked macronutrient, but it plays a crucial role in preventing many unwanted symptoms in the perimenopause body. Research consistently highlights the negative impact of a Western-style diet, which tends to be low in fibre and high in disease-promoting factors, including inflammation. All plant-based foods contain fibre with prebiotic effects. Prebiotic means the food nourishes the beneficial gut microbiome. A healthy gut microbiome is crucial for efficient nutrient absorption and the production of essential vitamins and precursor nutrients needed to create 'happy' neurotransmitters such as serotonin. Prebiotic foods also help gut microbiota produce anti-inflammatory compounds, which, in turn, can reduce inflammation throughout the body, including the brain. Studies suggest that inflammation may contribute to the development and persistence of conditions like depression and anxiety.

The *Mediterranean-style diet* stands out as an excellent choice during perimenopause and postmenopause. It is rich in fibre and prebiotic foods, and is considered one of the best diets for alleviating perimenopause/menopause symptoms. Epidemiological studies, which examine large groups of people, consistently show that those who consume more fibre tend to experience less weight gain, improved gut function, lower cancer rates, better mood, and reduced inflammation overall.

Fibre also aids in toxin removal from the body, preventing their reabsorption in the gut.

The UK NHS recommends a daily fibre intake of 30g. You can easily track your fibre consumption using food apps like MyNetDiary to become aware of your intake and identify areas for improvement. When increasing your fibre-rich foods, do so gradually to allow your gut to adapt and to avoid potential side effects like bloating, loose bowel movements or constipation.

Sources of fibre rich in prebiotics include vegetables, fruits, legumes, pulses, beans, nuts, seeds and whole grains. Some top choices for perimenopause and postmenopause due to their benefits include ground flax seeds, chia seeds, pumpkin seeds, raw almonds, lentils and chickpeas.

2. Unlocking the power of polyphenols

Polyphenols, the hidden gems found in all plant foods, are your allies in maintaining overall health and wellbeing. These potent plant compounds, varying with each type of plant food, have antioxidant and anti-inflammatory actions in the body. Plus, they nurture the beneficial gut microbiome, much like the role of fibre and prebiotics.

In return for eating polyphenol-rich plant food, the gut microbiota releases anti-inflammatory micronutrients that benefit your entire body. The synergy between polyphenols and your gut health can help alleviate the symptoms of perimenopause and menopause, making this knowledge a valuable asset in your journey to wellbeing.

Let's look at a few standouts:

- Green leafy vegetables, a polyphenol powerhouse. Green leafy vegetables, such as kale, chard, bok choy, choy sum, rocket, watercress, parsley and more, are rich sources of polyphenols. Take for example a group of polyphenols called carotenoids, found in many plant foods, including dark green leafy vegetables. They can act as strong antioxidants, boosting the body's own antioxidant defences. They have anti-diabetic effects, support collagen production and are useful for bone and cardiovascular health. Plus, there is some evidence that foods containing these bioactive carotenoids may decrease the risk of cancers such as oestrogen receptor-negative (ER-) breast cancer.

  All these green veggies are essential for your body and mind's overall health. In addition to polyphenols and fibre, they contain non-heme iron, B12, beta-carotene (a precursor to vitamin A), vitamin C, potassium, calcium, and other vital nutrients. Their role extends to hormone and mood balance, as well as bone health. Incorporating green leafy vegetables into your daily diet is a wise choice to support your wellbeing.

- Allicin vegetables, a gut- and liver-friendly choice. Vegetables in the allicin family, including onions, shallots, spring onions, leeks and garlic, are rich in polyphenols. The allicin vegetable family is known for its exceptional benefits for gut health and liver function. These vegetables help reduce inflammation, alleviate perimenopause symptoms, and even have a positive impact on cholesterol levels. Red onions and shallots boast high polyphenol levels of flavanols and anthocyanins, making them top choices for your health.

- Dark berries, Nature's polyphenol elixir. Dark berries such as blueberries, blackcurrants and blackberries are a treasure trove of polyphenols, including anthocyanins. These anthocyanin-rich polyphenols not only contribute to overall health but also enhance liver function. An efficiently functioning liver can potentially help alleviate perimenopause symptoms, such as low energy and mood, and hot flushes. Incorporate these dark berries into your diet to experience their multitude of benefits.

- Brassicas, which balance hormones with polyphenols. Brassica vegetables are another polyphenol-rich group known for their potential in balancing oestrogen levels. They contain a substance called di-indolyl-methane (DIM), which aids in the excretion of oestrogen after it has fulfilled its role. This property may help relieve associated issues like weight gain, mood swings, acne and perimenopause symptoms. Make it a habit to consume a serving or more of brassicas each day. The list includes broccoli, cauliflower, Brussels sprouts, cabbage, kale, swedes, turnips, asparagus and radishes, and various greens like bok choy, Chinese broccoli, choy sum and watercress.

- Cocoa, a delicious source of polyphenols. Embracing the power of polyphenols can be a delightful experience when you incorporate cocoa into your diet. Just one teaspoon of cocoa nibs added to your first meal of the day not only provides a rich source of polyphenols, but also supplies essential magnesium. Enjoy the satisfying crunch and the health benefits that come with it, making it a delicious addition to your breakfast routine.

3. Harnessing the power of phytoestrogens for your health

Phytoestrogens are Nature's gentle regulators found in a variety of plant-based foods. While not as potent as a woman's own oestrogen, they wield subtle but meaningful effects. They can lock on to and block the body's oestrogen receptors, protecting against the negative effects of too much-oestrogen, and conversely, they can also act as weak oestrogen signals on those same receptors when oestrogen is low.

Top sources of phytoestrogens include nuts, seeds, legumes and beans. Among these, flax seeds and chia seeds stand out for their high phytoestrogen lignan content. Soybeans, a potent source of phytoestrogens called isoflavones, reign supreme in the legume category. Research reveals that isoflavones from soy can alleviate hot flushes (approx. 80g firm tofu/day), reduce bone mineral density loss, enhance systolic blood pressure during early menopause and improve glycaemic control (blood sugar balance). In addition to their phytoestrogen content, nuts, seeds, legumes and beans offer a bounty of calcium and protein.

4. Fermented foods, your gut's best friend

Fermented foods, renowned for their anti-inflammatory benefits, play a crucial role in enhancing gut health. Live fermented foods contain beneficial microbes that collaborate with your gut microbiota to improve digestion and motility. Each fermented food boasts its unique strains of bacteria and yeasts, so experimentation is key. During perimenopause and postmenopause, when stress levels may rise, the gut microbiome can become out of balance and digestive enzyme production can decline. Fermented foods like sauerkraut, kimchi and live apple cider vinegar can stimulate digestive enzymes; thorough chewing also aids digestion. Other good, fermented options include dairy kefir, unsweetened live yogurt, kombucha, water kefir and nattō.

Note: If you have histamine intolerance, avoid fermented foods, unless you know you can tolerate them.

5. Omega-3 and other beneficial oils

Omega-3 oil is celebrated for its anti-inflammatory properties, which is especially welcome in perimenopause and menopause, when inflammation can increase, leading to an exacerbation in symptoms. The anti-inflammatory and health benefits come from the active converted forms of eicosapentaenoic acid (EPA) and docosahexaenoic acid (DHA). These active forms are found especially in oily fish, although all other seafood contains them but in lesser amounts. Plus, these active converted forms of EPA and DHA are also found in smaller amounts in sea vegetables/algae.

Alpha-linolenic acid (ALA), a precursor to EPA and DHA oils, is present in foods like soybeans, nuts and seeds, especially flax seeds, chia seeds and walnuts. Although the body struggles to convert ALA into active EPA and DHA, it manages to do so, albeit in modest quantities (around 8 per cent is converted). Extra virgin olive oil (EVOO) also provides anti-inflammatory benefits and contributes to alleviating perimenopause and menopause symptoms.

Fact: Did you know it is quite safe to cook with extra virgin olive oil?

6. The role of protein

Protein from your diet, once digested into amino acids, serves a multitude of functions in the body, including with oestrogen receptors. Regardless of the source – for example meat, seafood, diary or egg, or plant-based, like nuts and seeds such as hemp seeds and pistachio nuts – the body treats the resulting amino acids the same. Some prime plant protein sources with complete essential amino acids include quinoa, hemp seeds, pistachios and soy foods. Firm tofu boasts a high protein content, often rivalling that of salmon. As we age our body's ability to absorb and utilize protein becomes less efficient, so requirements from what you eat become higher.

Calculating your daily protein need is straightforward. Aim for 1.2g of protein per kilogram of body weight. For instance, a 70kg person would aim for approximately 84g of protein daily (the minimum requirement is 0.75g of protein per kilogram of body weight). Apps like MyNetDiary can help track your daily protein intake.

Additional considerations for optimal health

- Calcium is vital for bone strength, muscle function and mood regulation. The UK's NHS recommends calcium intake for an adult woman at 700mg per day. Dairy foods and soft edible fish bones are excellent sources. Nuts, seeds, and even some vegetables, such as green leafy vegetables and cabbage, and herbs contain calcium.
- Vitamin K works in tandem with calcium to build strong bones and is present in vegetables like parsley and broccoli and herbs such as basil and coriander. It is also found in fermented foods like sauerkraut.
- Vitamin D is found in modest amounts in oily fish, sunlight-exposed mushrooms and fortified foods. Vitamin D is crucial for bone health, inflammation reduction, neuromuscular function, immune health and glucose metabolism. Supplements are often recommended for sufficient intake.
- Magnesium, which is generally low in the foods we eat, is important for reducing inflammation, affecting a wide range of symptoms such as cognitive impairment, depression, metabolic disease, sarcopenia and osteoporosis.
- B vitamins are important for energy production, bone health, processing of carbohydrates and the functioning of the nervous system.
- Sea vegetables (also known as seaweed) are rich in iodine, zinc and

prebiotic soluble fibre. Iodine is essential for thyroid function, impacting metabolism, weight and energy levels.

What doesn't help?

- Sugar and refined carbohydrates, which are devoid of fibre and essential nutrients, lead to inflammation, gut microbiome depletion, calcium loss from bones, type 2 diabetes and mood imbalances. If eating grains, opt for complex, unrefined grains like whole rolled oats, buckwheat, spelt and quinoa.
- Limit saturated, trans and hydrogenated fats to reduce headaches, menstrual cramps, endometriosis discomfort and perimenopause symptoms. Diets high in saturated fats hinder the absorption of essential fats from foods like nuts, seeds, avocado and olive oil.
- Be mindful of caffeine, which may cause anxiety, blood glucose spikes and hot flushes during perimenopause. Excessive caffeine depletes essential minerals and vitamins and exacerbates perimenopausal symptoms.
- Alcohol affects perimenopause and postmenopause symptoms, and can contribute to blood sugar imbalance, weight gain, and gut, bone and mental health issues.
- Smoking affects perimenopause and postmenopause symptoms, and can contribute to cardiovascular, bone and gut health issues.

Note: Incorporating these polyphenol- and fibre-rich foods into your diet can make a significant difference in managing inflammation and gut health, and the symptoms associated with perimenopause and menopause. However, always consult with your healthcare provider before making substantial dietary changes, especially if you have any underlying medical condition(s) or concerns. Your journey towards wellbeing can be both delicious and rewarding with the right choices in your diet.

You can download Emma's recipes from her website, Emma's Nutrition.*

Emma Ellice Flint, BHSc nutritionist & author

---

* www.emmasnutrition.com

Herbal remedies

Herbal remedies have been taken for hundreds of years, and many of our modern medicines were originally based on plant extracts. The British Menopause Society (BMS) recommends using some herbal remedies that have been subjected to scientific research and proven beneficial. However, it is essential that you seek the guidance of a qualified herbalist, that the herbs are from a trusted source, and that you stick to the advised dosage. If you are taking prescription medication, have had hormone receptor cancer or are taking HRT, please check with your doctor or medical herbalist before you start taking herbal remedies. Some herbs, such as black cohosh, can interfere with other medications, and phytoestrogens are not currently recommended for women with hormone receptor cancer.

Here, medical herbalist Melinda McDougall gives us an overview of herbal remedies for menopausal symptoms.

People always ask me: 'What's the one herb I can take for menopause?' If only it were that simple. We are all different and our individual experiences of menopause will vary greatly. A typical prescription I create for someone from my dispensary will contain around seven different liquid plant extracts, working on many different aspects of treatment. No one is 'just' a menopausal woman – I'm sure you'll agree that there's a lot going on at this time of life – mentally, emotionally and physically.

You might be experiencing symptoms like hot flushes, heavy periods, insomnia, anxiety and a sense of being overwhelmed – the list can feel endless. But it doesn't have to be all doom and gloom. While it can be challenging for all of us, I'm always excited to see how the women I work with can harness the energy of this transitional time to change their lives and their health for the better.

Herbal medicine has been used by women for hundreds of years to support their health during menopause. It comes in many forms – teas, tinctures (liquids), capsules and powders. Always buy from reputable sources – cheap menopause supplements often contain little in the way of active herbs. In the UK, looking for the traditional herbal registration (THR) logo is a good place to start.

Liquid extracts, or tinctures, are my favourite way of working with herbal medicines. They are potent, effective and only require small doses, usually taken twice daily. Don't underestimate the power of a strong cup of loose-leaf herbal tea though.

Here are some of my favourite herbal remedies for menopausal symptoms – herbs that I use in clinical practice every day:

- Hot flushes and night sweats: sage (*salvia officinalis*), black cohosh (*actaea racemosa*), wild yam (*dioscorea villosa*).
- Erratic menstrual cycles and premenstrual syndrome (PMS): chaste tree berry (*vitex agnus-castus*).
- Heavy periods can be very debilitating during perimenopause (always make sure other gynaecological causes such as fibroids are ruled out and check your iron levels): Lady's mantle (*alchemilla vulgaris*), yarrow (*achillea millefolium*), nettle (*urtica dioica*) and shepherd's purse (*capsella bursa-pastoris*) are a great combination, working in synergy to stem the heavy flow.
- Anxiety, rage and mood swings: St John's wort (*hypericum perforatum*), rose (*rosa damascena*), blue skullcap (*scutellaria lateriflora*).
- Brain fog: gotu kola (*centella asiatica*), gingko (*ginkgo biloba*).
- Stress and burnout: You may have heard of 'adaptogens'. This is a class of herbs that help our bodies 'adapt' to stress. They are crucial in menopause as we go through the transition. Ashwaganda (*withania somnifera*) helps us to feel calm while rhodiola (*rhodiola rosea*) can help with mental focus and Siberian ginseng (*eleutherococcus senticosus*) is useful for energy and immune support.
- Insomnia: valerian (*valeriana officinalis*), passionflower (*passiflora incarnata*), blue skullcap (*scutellaria lateriflora*).
- Liver support: This is crucial for healthy metabolism of hormones. As well as taking herbs, support your liver function by drinking plenty of water and reducing caffeine, processed foods and alcohol. Dandelion root (*taraxacum officinale radix*) and milk thistle (*silybum marianum*) help support healthy liver function during menopause.
- Low libido: shatavari (*asparagus racemosus*), maca root (*lepidium meyenii*).

- Vaginal dryness: shatavari (*asparagus racemosus*), sea buckthorn oil (*hippophae rhamnoides*).[2]

Melinda McDougall, MSc, MNIMH, menopause
specialist and medical herbalist. You can download
Melinda's free guide to herbal medicine and menopause
from her website: www.melindamcdougall.com.

AYURVEDA

Ayurveda is a holistic system of healthcare that originated in the Indian subcontinent and is still used today to treat the whole person (mind and body). This Sanskrit word *Ayur-veda* means science of life and views dis-ease as the result of an imbalance, which can be brought back to equilibrium (sattva) through specific foods, herbal remedies, yoga (poses, meditation, breathing) and massage. Here are some of the ayurvedic remedies that may help you manage some of your menopause symptoms. One of the most popular is ashwaganda because it is an adaptogen, meaning that it can help us adapt to change. The perimenopause to postmenopause transition is one of the biggest times of change, so try this first and see if you feel any benefits. Each of us is unique, however, so it is important to seek the advice of an Ayurveda practitioner.

Here is some general guidance from Ayurvedic practitioner Deena Solanki.

- Aloe vera juice aids digestion and has a cooling effect to balance all doshas.
- Ashwagandha is an adaptogenic herb that calms stress, builds mental strength and promotes sleep.
- Dashamula reduces pain and inflammation in the pelvic and sacral area, directs vata downwards and supports the nervous system.
- Kaishore guggulu reduces inflammation in joints and muscles.
- Liquorice clears ama* from the gut and may support the endocrine system, especially the adrenal gland.

---

* *Āma* is an Ayurvedic term that indicates 'the abnormal or impaired process of digestion and metabolism that leads to build up of toxic by-products, which cannot be neutralized or eliminated by the body. Manohar PR. Critical review and validation of the concept of Āma. Anc Sci Life. 2012 Oct;32(2):67-8. doi: 10.4103/0257-7941.118524. PMID: 24167329; PMCID: PMC3807959.

- Shatavari is a strengthening herb that can feel cooling. It contains phytoestrogens and regulates hormones, enhances libido, calms the nervous system, and is mildly diuretic.
- Triphala maintains a healthy digestive tract, and helps reduce constipation, sluggish digestion and bloating. It is cooling for all doshas.
- Turmeric reduces inflammation.
- Usheera can reduce excess heat, burning sensations and sweating.
- Yogaraja guggulu is a muscle relaxant that helps ease painful menstruation.

Deena Solanki, an Ayurvedic practitioner

Self-massage with oils (abhyanga)

The ancient Ayurvedic therapy of self-massage (abhyanga) from head to toe using warm essential oils has many benefits for men and women at any age, but in menopause it can be one of the most nourishing, healing acts of self-love and care. Ayurveda recommends different oils for different constitutions or doshas.

The physical benefits of self-massage with oils are said to be:

- Moisturizing your skin, hair and nails, which become dryer in menopause
- Lubricating your joints (which may help with frozen shoulder and other joint pain)
- Easing muscle pain
- Stimulating blood circulation
- Arousing libido
- Supporting lymphatic drainage
- Calming anxiety, lifting low mood and fatigue
- Relaxing you for sleep.

HOW TO SELF-MASSAGE, STEP BY STEP

1. Choose your oil for a specific effect and warm it in a cup (do not use hot oil as it could burn your skin).
2. Pour a little oil on the crown of your head and massage your scalp in a circular motion, including your hair roots (avoid your eyes).
3. Massage your face using upward strokes, including your ear lobes.

4. Massage your arms and legs with long strokes towards your heart.

5. Massage your abdomen to aid digestion, using circular movements from the right hip bone, up and around to the left hip bone. This follows the route of your digestion in the ascending and descending colon.

6. Massage your feet and allow time for the oil to be absorbed.

7. Relax for 15 minutes before having a shower, but avoid using detergents or soaps as this will wash away the moisturizing oil. Pat your skin dry.

Exercise

Modern life is too sedentary; it is linked to increasing health risks and may be contributing to your menopause symptoms. Physical movement has been proven to reduce the risk of cardiovascular disease, diabetes and dementia, it can improve mental health and may help manage weight gain. Research shows it may also alleviate menopause symptoms, including anxiety, insomnia, restless leg syndrome, low mood and lethargy, bloating and sluggish digestion, and help you to maintain muscle and bone strength, which weaken as oestrogen declines.

TYPES OF EXERCISE

Different forms of exercise or movement have different benefits, so it is important to vary your physical activity and adapt your exercise to your daily needs. For example:

- Flexibility and mobility: yoga, swimming, Pilates, walking.
- Calming anxiety: yoga and swimming, gentle running.
- Lifting low mood: strength training and aerobic exercise such as dancing and Zumba.
- Balance and coordination: yoga, qigong and tai chi.
- Bone and muscle strength: lifting weights, resistance training, running.
- Heart health and diabetes: aerobic movement, yoga to reduce stress.

Adapting exercise to menopause stages

It is important to adapt the pace and length of your activity for different stages of premenopause to postmenopause:

- Premenopause. On average, your mid-to late 30s is when your OPT hormones start to gradually decline. This is a good time to prepare for perimenopause by strengthening muscles, bones and cardiovascular health, which will both help you manage psychological symptoms that start to arise (anxiety, overwhelm, mood swings) and help reduce your risk of osteoporosis and sarcopenia, etc.

- Perimenopause. On average this will be in your mid-to late 40s, when your OPT hormones are fluctuating and you may miss or have shorter or longer menstrual periods. This can be an emotionally and physically exhausting time that lasts from three to seven years or more. Your body and brain are working hard to bring you back to balance, so if you overload yourself with stress and excessive exercise, believing you can power through the symptoms, then you're likely to end up exhausted and burnt out, which causes negative stress. The unpredictable peaks and troughs in your OPT hormones mean you may feel able to run a marathon one day and unable to get out of bed the next. The decline in oestrogen may cause inflammation in your joints and muscles, so this is the time to slow down and listen to your body to avoid getting injured. Swimming, gentle somatic and vinyasa flow yoga, walking, and being in Nature are ideal. Pilates can also help maintain core muscle strength, as well as recovery after injury.

- Menopause. On average, this is in your early 50s, and is medically defined as 12 months without a menstrual bleed, although it can last longer. This is a time for you to *pause* and go inward as your body and brain, in their innate wisdom, are adapting to the permanent change in your hormones. Instead of sourcing oestradiol from your ovaries, your adrenal glands kick in and can convert some adipose fatty tissues into a lower grade oestrone. This can help ease some of your symptoms so you need to rest, do less and reduce stress, to avoid overloading your endocrine system. This is a time to practise restorative and somatic yoga, meditation and deep rest in yoga nidra. Qigong, swimming and being in Nature, earthing (walking barefoot on grass) or forest bathing can be grounding too.

- Postmenopause. The new STRAW definition[3] says you may still become pregnant three years after your final menstrual bleed. Medically we know that the sharpest decline in these hormones is for five years after menopause, which is why you may notice the sharpest fall in bone density and muscle mass. To prevent this, you can start using you own body weight to build strength and protect your long-term health and happiness. Feeling stronger feels good! We are not weak and feeble; our bodies and brains want to bounce back. Start gently with the yoga for strength, balance, etc. classes in this book (see 'MY class for balance', and 'MY class for strength'), using your own body weight and resistance bands as well as Pilates. You need core muscle strength to support your lower back (lumbar spine, tailbone and sacroiliac joint) as well as other joints, and to avoid sciatica and muscle strain.

- Second Spring. As you build self-confidence you can add some weights to your yoga practice and start joining strength training classes. Menopause changes our sensitivity to noise, overstim-ulation and crowded places, so you may find a loud, busy HIIT (high-intensity interval training) class at a gym is not right for you. I advise you to seek the professional guidance of a fitness instructor before using heavy weights. Once you get started, you may surprise yourself with how much weight you can lift, and how good it feels to feel strong.

Strength training

Lavina Mehta, MBE, is a personal trainer and wellness coach who campaigns for making movement accessible through the concept of 'exercise snacking' – short movement sessions that you can easily fit into your day that may last a few minutes, 15 minutes or up to half an hour, if that feels good for you. In her book, *The Feel Good Fix: Boost Energy, Improve Sleep and Move More Through Menopause and Beyond*, Mehta extols the benefits of exercise, especially strength training, to maintain muscle strength that depletes after menopause (sarcopenia), boost bone density that declines as we age (osteopenia and osteoporosis), joint mobility and balance (to avoid falls and bone fractures), as well as improvements in supporting your heart and mental health.

Regular strength training can also help you maintain a healthy body weight (body fat often accumulates around your midriff – the 'menopot' – which may increase the risk of cardiovascular health). Lean muscle burns off more calories than adipose (fat) tissues, so your metabolism becomes more efficient. Maintaining a healthy weight may also reduce the risk of heart disease, dementia and type 2 diabetes.

What is strength training?

You can practise strength training using your own body weight and progress to lifting hand and machine gym weights. Over time, you will gain even more strength from 'progressive loading' where you exert more physical stress on your bones and muscles. According to the LIFTMOR study in 2018,[4] high-intensity resistance and impact training (HiRIT) can help women in postmenopause who have low bone density, especially if you increase the load or weights you lift. Did you know that our bones get bored if we plateau and just stick with the same regime? So, for the best results, vary the exercises and weights to keep your body and brain stimulated in a positive, healthy way.

Please note: If you have osteoporosis, then you need to seek the professional guidance of your doctor and physiotherapist to tailor the weights and exercises to your individual needs.

Myokines and strength training

Myokines are natural chemicals released from your muscles when you exercise. Research suggests that myokines can boost your metabolism, support balanced blood sugar levels, are anti-inflammatory, and improve your brain function and mental health. Lavina Mehta says: 'When you exercise, your body naturally pushes myokines out of your muscles. They then enter the blood stream and cross over the blood-brain barrier, acting as anti-depressants. Therefore, when people exercise, they feel better.'[5]

In Menopause Yoga we include strength training that uses body weight. However, I also offer the option to include hand weights in specific poses such as chair pose and goddess squats for an extra boost of physical and brain energy, which can also lift your mood as well as strengthen your muscles. (See 'MY class for strength' for a 5-, 15- and 30-minute class you can fit into your day.)

Nature

A growing body of research shows that being outdoors in Nature reduces both physical and psychological stress levels for those visitors to a natural environment. Earthing (walking barefoot on grass) and forest bathing (lying down in a wood or forest) are increasingly popular for stress relief, and the colour green has been linked to feelings of relaxation.[6]

COLD WATER SWIMMING

During my perimenopause, when I had muscle and joint inflammation and could barely walk, the one thing I could do was swim, or at least float and let the water hold me. The cold water eased the inflammation – and I could move again without pain.

Cold water swimming in the UK has recently become very popular among menopausal women cooling their hot flushes in the sea. Research by University College London (UCL) in 2024 suggests that menopausal women experience a significant improvement in anxiety (as reported by 46.9 per cent of the women), mood swings (34.5 per cent), low mood (31.1 per cent) and hot flushes (30.3 per cent) as a result of cold water swimming.[7] In addition, a majority of the women (63.3 per cent) swam specifically to relieve their symptoms.

Some said that they found the cold water to be 'an immediate stress/ anxiety reliever' and described the activity as 'healing'. One 57-year-old woman stated: 'Cold water is phenomenal. It has saved my life. In the water, I can do anything. All symptoms (physical and mental) disappear, and I feel like me at my best.'[8]

Professor Joyce Harper, UCL EGA Institute for Women's Health says:

Looking after our lifestyle is key throughout our lives but becomes even more important during the perimenopause and beyond. Three important factors are exercise, mental health and community and friendships. There is growing research data that shows that just being outside improves our mental health, so if you add to this exercising with friends, it is a win: win. And I would add one more dimension to this – being near or in water. In my research, many people tell me that being near water is their happy place. For many years I have been a cold water swimmer and it makes me very happy, and helps my mental health. I was aware that many people who swim are women around perimenopause age.

I embarked on a study to ask more women about cold water swimming and menstrual and menopause symptoms. Our research at UCL showed that women certainly felt cold water swimming reduced their menstrual and perimenopause symptoms and we are doing more studies into this. They rated the effects of the cold water as the main reason why they thought it helped them. I really love being outside, looking at a beautiful view, being surrounded by Nature, getting into cool water and swimming with a group of women who make me laugh. It is such a great hobby and it is so good for us, though we do need to careful and responsible in cold water. Always swim with others.

Professor Joyce Harper, UCL EGA Institute for Women's Health

Talking therapies and cognitive behavioural therapy

I realized I had packed my emotional store cupboard with unprocessed emotions. At perimenopause, the store cupboard door flew open and tumbled out. It felt like a mess, but talking therapy helped me make sense of these memories – I was able to heal. It was like a good spring clean! I was able to sort through the mess, let go of what I no longer needed and choose what I wanted to put back into the cupboard. (Petra Coveney)

MENTAL HEALTH

Menopause can have a significant impact on a woman's emotional well-being. While some may embrace the end of their menstrual cycle and experience few difficulties, others face challenges. During perimenopause, fluctuating hormone levels – especially oestrogen, progesterone and testosterone – can heighten vulnerability to emotional and mental health issues. Neuroscientist Dr Mosconi notes that these hormonal shifts can rewire the brain, leading to anxiety, low mood, depression or trauma-related symptoms, whether from past events or the transition itself. During this time, talking therapies can be valuable in processing emotions, helping women navigate menopause and embrace their 'Second Spring'. All talking therapies can be beneficial, with the British and International Menopause Societies specifically endorsing cognitive behavioural therapy (CBT) for its effectiveness and evidence-based approach.

COGNITIVE BEHAVIOURAL THERAPY

CBT is a widely recognized approach for treating emotional, psychological and mental health issues. It serves as an umbrella term for various cognitive and behavioural therapies. Traditional CBT focuses on challenging unhelpful thoughts to improve emotional wellbeing, while newer forms emphasize changing how we relate to difficult thoughts, encouraging actions that align with our core values and what matters most to us as individuals.

In Part Four: Daily Practices, I have included some of the CBT techniques that I use in Menopause Yoga classes for specific symptoms. Some are informed by the British Menopause Society's (BMS) recommended CBT, and some are my own techniques based on ancient yoga philosophy explained in the Yoga Sutras of Patanjali. One of these is pratipaksha bhavana (choosing to view a difficult situation from an opposite perspective in order to change how you feel). I hope you find them helpful.

However, if you find the emotional and psychological changes are too much to handle on your own, please seek professional support from a qualified mental health professional. This is not a sign of weakness; it is a positive action of self-care, and may give you the opportunity to resolve issues in a healthy way. CBT is just one form of taking therapies, and you may prefer a different approach. The key to successful therapy is finding the right therapist for your needs. Take your time, reach out to a few options, and choose thoughtfully.

A good benchmark is selecting a therapist accredited by a professional body who offers a menopause-informed approach, like psychologist Simona Stokes.

Third-wave CBT approaches, like acceptance and commitment therapy (ACT), compassion focused therapy (CFT) and others, can be especially effective for managing the psychological and emotional challenges of menopause. Rather than trying to change or eliminate difficult thoughts and emotions, these therapies focus on creating distance between you and your thoughts, fostering acceptance of all emotions, cultivating self-compassion, and encouraging actions that align with your core values.

This is my EMBERS® model, which is based on third-wave CBT approaches and has been specially tailored for menopause. It considers the hormonal context and provides a holistic framework to address physical, psychological and external life challenges encountered during menopause, empowering women to navigate this transition with resilience and confidence.

Try this self-reflection exercise.

Transforming suffering into coping
Objective

This exercise aims to help you transition from suffering to coping by fostering awareness of the processes involved. Suffering often arises from a lack of understanding of our physical, emotional and cognitive changes, leading to misinterpretations of symptoms and increased anxiety. Common responses include rejecting and resisting these experiences, often resorting to impulsive behaviours that provide only temporary relief.

To move towards coping, it is essential to cultivate awareness and acceptance, allowing emotions to surface as messages about unmet needs. Practising self-compassion and aligning actions with core values – such as curiosity, love and kindness – enables thoughtful responses to challenges. Ultimately, this shift empowers individuals to navigate life's difficulties more effectively and promotes a more fulfilling experience.

Instructions

1. Reflect on your symptoms:
   - Take a moment to identify any physical or emotional symptoms you are currently experiencing (e.g., anxiety, fatigue, heart palpitations).
   - Write down your thoughts on what you believe is causing these symptoms. Are you attributing them to stress, personal issues or something else?

2. Explore mislabelling:
   - Reflect on whether you might be misinterpreting your symptoms.
   - Write down any assumptions you have about these feelings. Are you viewing them as signs of weakness or a serious problem?

3. Acknowledge your emotions:
   - Allow yourself to sit with your emotions. Write about how you feel without judgement.
   - Consider what these emotions might be telling you about your unmet needs or conflicted values.

4. Practise self-compassion:
   - Write a compassionate note to yourself, acknowledging your feelings and offering support.
   - Remind yourself that it's okay to feel what you're feeling and that you are not alone in this experience.

5. Identify core values:
   - Reflect on what truly matters to you in life (e.g., family, health, career, self-care).
   - Write down your core values and consider how they influence your decisions and actions.

6. Align actions with values:
   - Think of one or two small actions you can take that align with your core values.
   - Write down these actions and commit to implementing them in your daily life (e.g., setting aside time for self-care, reaching out to a friend).

7. Evaluate your progress:
   - After a week, revisit this exercise. Reflect on any changes you noticed in your feelings, behaviours or overall wellbeing.
   - Write down your observations and consider what you learned about yourself during this process.

Closing reflection: Take a few minutes to sit quietly and reflect on your journey. Acknowledge the progress you've made in shifting from suffering to coping, and remind yourself that this is an ongoing process. Celebrate your efforts and commitment to your wellbeing.

Simona Stokes, psychologist and creator of EMBERS®
menopause-informed CBT framework

---

* www.menopausecbtclinic.co.uk/embers

Journaling

Journaling is the gateway to self-knowledge and self-growth.

The most important relationship we can all have is the one you have with yourself, the most important journey you can take is one of self-discovery. To know yourself, you must spend time with yourself, you must not be afraid to be alone. Knowing yourself is the beginning of all wisdom. (Aristotle, approx. 350 BCE)

Keeping a journal is valuable during your perimenopause to menopause transition. A journal/diary can become a companion who helps you download anxious thoughts, chew through troublesome feelings to find solutions, and track your symptoms linked to what you eat or drink, activities such as exercise or work, and relationships and conversations that impact your levels of stress and sleep. It will also make a great read when you are on the other side.

Here is some general advice on keeping a journal, but remember, it does not have to be words; you can record on your phone or draw pictures and diagrams.

I have noticed themes appearing in my journal – negative thoughts towards myself and fear/resisting the menopause and getting older. I have been scared for quite some time about my menopause journey and actively resisted it. I realize I have taken on board what society and the media think about older women and the menopause. I now want to be part of a generation that normalize the topic of menopause for men and women. Acceptance and empowerment are key words in my journal.

I write when I first wake up and I am noticing it is helping me prepare for the day ahead. I notice my thoughts, but don't attach labels to them as good or bad.

Kat Aydin, yoga teacher

CREATING NEW HABITS

Journaling can help you create new habits by:

- Observing objectively. Use journaling as a meditation technique to tune into your emotions for the day. Ask yourself: 'What am I feeling today? Where am I feeling it and why? What do I need? Can I give this to myself?'
- Self-reflection. Journaling prompts like 'What is it that I need to let go of?' or 'What is holding me back from living a happier, healthier life?' can spark self-reflection and open the door to inner awareness.

JOURNALING AS A TOOL FOR CHANGE

Journaling offers a powerful tool for managing mental health and navigating change during menopause.

Daily journal

- Track food and drink. List what you eat and drink without judgement. Note the timing of meals.
- Record your physical, mental and emotional state. Reflect on how you felt throughout the day (physically, mentally and emotionally). Did the food nourish you?
- Activities. List your daily activities (exercise, work, socializing, hobbies).
- Sleep patterns. Track your sleep schedule, noting sleep quality, disturbances and wake-up times.
- Journaling frequency. Record when you journal (before bed, in the morning or during the night).
- Morning reflections. Reflect on your physical, mental and emotional state on waking up.

By tracking this information, you can identify patterns and connections that might trigger your symptoms, empowering you to make informed choices for your wellbeing.

Different journaling styles

- Reflective journaling. Regularly reflect on your life, needs and wants. Prompts can be helpful (e.g., Where am I now? Where do I want to be? Why?).
- Affirmations. Focus on positive self-talk related to relationships, finances or health. Start affirmations with 'I am' (e.g., I am strong, I am supported).
- Intentions. Ask yourself questions to identify your needs (e.g., What does my soul need today? How do I want to feel?).
- Scripting. Visualize your ideal future in detail, describing your surroundings, sensations and emotions.
- Gratitude journaling. List things you're grateful for, such as someone's actions, your achievements or simple pleasures.
- Dream journaling.

Journal reflection prompts

- Past reflections:
  - What brought you happiness and fulfilment in life?
  - What held you back from achieving your dreams?
  - Is there anyone you need to forgive to move forward?

- Present day:
  - How can you accept yourself completely?
  - What gives you purpose, and is it changing?
  - If moving to a new place, what would you bring (and leave behind)?

- Future dreams and desires:
  - What are your dreams and desires?
  - How can you find your voice and express yourself?

If you like journals, you will love *The Perimenopause Journal* written by Kate Codrington, which includes season tackers and beautiful illustrations.

LIFESTYLE WELLBEING CHECKLIST

- Prioritize yourself. Learn to say *yes* to yourself and *no* to others.
- Reduce stress and inflammation. Learn stress management techniques to lower inflammation and improve overall health: yoga, breathwork and meditation.
- Rest and restore your energy. Get enough sleep and nap when you need.
- Nourish yourself. Eat warm cooked foods, include plant-based phytoestrogens, calcium and vitamins D, C and K to maintain bone density. Reduce salt and sugar, alcohol, caffeine, processed foods and unhealthy fats.
- Hydrate. Drink plenty of water.
- Exercise snacks to boost balance, bones, brain and heart health – avoid burnout.
- 'Exercise snacks' are short bouts of vigorous exercise performed throughout the day in order to improve health and wellbeing.'[9]
- Strength and resistance training can reduce long-term health risks.
- Nurture yourself. Practise self-compassion and prioritize self-care, e.g., massage.
- Nature. Qigong, forest bathing, earthing (barefoot walking on grass) and cold water swimming.
- Stay connected. Socialize – don't isolate yourself.
- Talk to friends, family, your doctor or a counsellor.
- Journaling. Track your symptoms, gain insights, and include daily gratitude and joy.
- Embrace change. Let go of what no longer serves you and move forward with a renewed perspective. Embrace your Second Spring.
- Daily routine. Wake up with dawn, go to bed at 10pm and eat at set times of the day; eat earlier in the evening so there is time to digest food, and avoid skipping meals.
- Avoid multitasking. Allow yourself time to focus on one 'job' at a time.

Part Three

YOGA BASICS

Menopause Yoga isn't a magic pill; it's a holistic whole-person health-care approach that can work alongside medical and lifestyle changes. (Petra Coveney)

In this part I'll introduce you to some of the various strands of the Menopause Yoga practice and some techniques for each one: breathwork (pranayama), mudras and mantras and yoga nidra. Read through these sections carefully, watch the videos using the QR codes, and then try them for yourself.

Yoga health benefits

Yoga is a mind – body integrated approach to health that can help you through menopause alongside other lifestyle and medical support. Widespread international research[1] shows yoga can help alleviate symptoms of polycystic ovary syndrome (PCOS) and menopause, although the studies are often small. The latest studies from the All India Institute of Medical Sciences (AIIMS), in New Delhi, India, confirm that yoga can even help to prevent long-term health risks.

Dr Rima Dada, from the All India Institute of Medical Sciences, New Delhi (AIIMS), says that practising yoga daily has been shown to lower chronic inflammation, caused by high oxidative and psychological stress levels, which could help reduce depression and anxiety, and reduce the risk of developing metabolic syndrome, PCOS, Alzheimer's disease, depression, cancer and autoimmune diseases. Research by Dr Dada's group found that a regular practice of yoga can reduce our biological age, and we can enjoy not only a longer lifespan but also a longer health span. In addition, yoga helps to normalize hormonal levels, regulate immune ageing and improve both mitochondrial and nuclear DNA integrity.[2]

In an article for this book, Dr Dada says:

Our research found that yoga helps to reduce levels of the stress hormone cortisol by regulating our sympathetic nervous system which controls the stress response. High and chronic (long-term) inflammation is linked to a wide range of health issues from cancer, dementia to diabetes, and stiff joints, and decline in mental health. Yoga builds emotional resilience by promoting neuroplasticity.[3]

MENTAL HEALTH AND EMOTIONAL WELLBEING

As we learned in Part One, lower levels of oestrogen (and progesterone) can make it harder for your brain to produce mood-regulating chemicals: serotonin, noradrenaline, oxytocin and dopamine. Yoga, meditation and breathing exercises cannot replace these hormones or brain chemicals, but they can help regulate your mental health by:

- Reducing stress and inflammation
- Improving sleep
- Aiding digestion
- Alleviating mood swings
- Enhancing mental focus.

PHYSICAL HEALTH

Yoga can help reduce stress and inflammation, potentially alleviating some of these menopausal side effects and long-term health risks listed in Part One.[4] It can also benefit muscles, cardiovascular health and lungs.[5] The flexibility and mobility benefits of yoga can keep you moving, allowing you to stay socially connected and take up other forms of strength-building exercise.

What is Menopause Yoga?

Menopause Yoga is a holistic approach because the menopause affects the whole person: mind, body, and emotions.

Menopause Yoga draws on ancient yoga philosophy (Patanjali's Yoga Sutras) that encourages people to accept change as a natural, normal part of living, so that we learn to relax into rather than resist the menopause. Although Menopause Yoga cannot replace or rebalance the hormones that decline in menopause, it can support you in this significant life transition. As in Indian Ayurveda, Menopause Yoga *does not* see the menopause as a disease, sickness or syndrome. It is viewed as a time of imbalance caused by fluctuating hormones that may manifest as dis-ease in your mind, body and emotions.

Yoga is a tool of Ayurveda to help bring you back to ease or balance. Imbalance will affect each person differently because you are unique. For some people the imbalance may show up as specific symptoms that reflect the doshas, for example hot flushes (pitta), bloating (vata) and weight gain (kapha). Or the imbalance may reflect our energies (the gunas) that make us mentally overactive (rajas) or depressed (tamas). The aim of the yoga practice is to bring you back to a state of equilibrium (sattva), because this is your place of optimal physical health and mental wellbeing.

Menopause Yoga is a specialized practice that, like pregnancy yoga, offers specific techniques:

- Symptom relief. Poses, breathing and meditation techniques aim to ease common menopause symptoms.
- Positive mindset. Reframing menopause as a positive transition can improve overall wellbeing. We call it our Second Spring.
- Modifications. Practices are modified according to menopause

symptoms and adjusted for individual needs (e.g., avoiding deep bends for osteoporosis).

- Journaling. Tracking your symptoms and emotional journey gives you a valuable insight into personal triggers that could change your life and lifestyle.
- Community. In-person classes connect you with others experiencing menopause.

Overall, Menopause Yoga helps navigate menopause with a focus on self-care, empowerment and a renewed sense of self-confidence.

YOGA THERAPY: WESTERN SCIENCE AND EASTERN TRADITIONS

As a yoga therapist, I created Menopause Yoga to give you a therapeutic approach to your individual needs. It views symptoms as signs of internal imbalances in energy flow, mental states and physical wellbeing, combining Western medical science and Eastern models (Indian Ayurveda and Traditional Chinese Medicine). While Western medical practitioners specialize in anatomy, psychology, physiology, gynaecology etc., separating the body and brain and emotions, both Ayurveda and TCM view you holistically (mind, body, spirit). These are different prisms to view the same person but can be combined to support your individual needs.

This book is not a substitute for one-on-one support with a qualified yoga therapist, but I hope my positive holistic approach, classes and videos can be a great starting point.

TIME OF DAY

This section explores the optimal times to practise Menopause Yoga throughout the day and during your menstrual cycle.

Morning: Boost digestion and balance cortisol

- Ideally, practise yoga postures (asanas) in the morning, before breakfast and caffeine.

- An empty stomach, from overnight fasting, allows yoga to stimulate digestion in preparation for food.
- Menopause can slow metabolism, so this 'morning practice' helps 'stoke the digestive fire'.
- Morning cortisol, a hormone that wakes you up, naturally increases with daylight.
- A short (15-minute) morning practice can help balance cortisol levels, stretch your limbs and set a positive tone for the day.

Afternoon: Rest and recharge

- Feeling fatigued in the afternoon? Try a restorative pose for 10–15 minutes.
- If desk work leaves you stiff or sluggish, practise energizing breaths and movements.
- Examples of energizing practices include bellows breath, skull shining breath, breath of joy, chair pose, goddess pose and meno-warrior squats. These practices can boost your heart rate and improve brain focus.
- Avoid napping in the afternoon in bed. This may mess up your natural circadian rhythm. Keep your bedroom for sleep at night.

Evening: Unwind

- An evening wind-down class helps release muscle tension accumulated throughout the day.
- Spinal flexibility stretches decompress your spine, promoting relaxation.
- Forward folds to stretch the back of your legs, a bridge pose or full body stretch both help to stimulate your yawn response which tones your vagus nerve and helps prepare you for sleep.

Nighttime: Gentle preparation for sleep

- A nighttime gentle practice includes a restorative inversion such as legs raised against the wall pose, designed to prepare you for sleep.

KEY TAKEAWAY

Listen to your body and choose the practice time that best suits your energy levels and needs. A 5- to 10-minute practice daily is better than 90 minutes once a week.

MENSTRUAL CYCLE CONSIDERATIONS

- Your menstrual cycle has phases with varying hormone levels.
- Follicle-stimulating hormone (FSH) and oestradiol help release an egg, while luteinizing hormone (LH) and progesterone prepare the womb for pregnancy.
- Decreasing hormone levels trigger menstruation (period).
- These hormonal fluctuations affect your body temperature and energy levels, and may cause symptoms like headaches, bloating, sore breasts, mood swings and food cravings. These fluctuations can impact your exercise effectiveness.

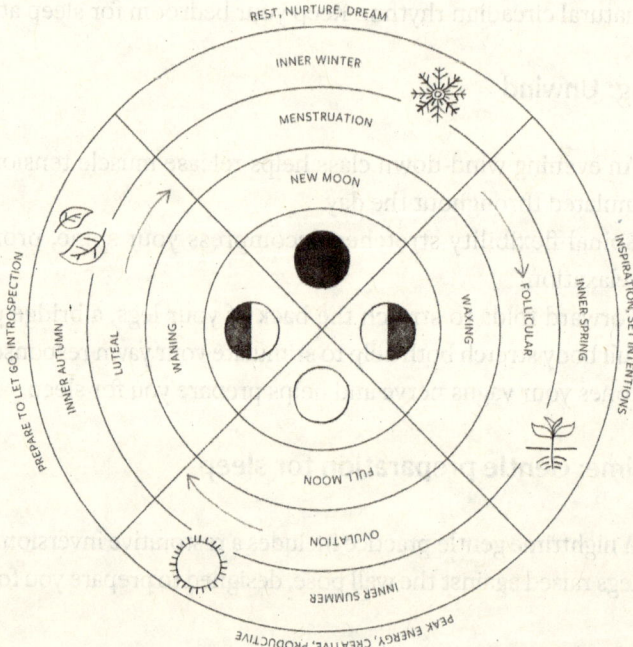

PHASES AND CYCLES

Understanding your yoga needs through your cycle

This section explains how your menstrual cycle and hormonal changes can impact your ideal yoga practice.

PHASES OF YOUR MENSTRUAL CYCLE
Phase 1: Follicular stage (Inner Spring/Waxing Moon)

- Follicle-stimulating hormone (FSH) increases, leading to ovulation and oestrogen production.
- You have more energy and a more positive mood and motivation to set goals.

Ideal yoga: Uplifting morning classes to benefit from oestrogen-fuelled flexibility. Consider grounding and calming practices in the evening to promote sleep.

Phase 2: Ovulation stage (Inner Summer/Full Moon)

- Peak oestrogen levels lead to peak energy and endurance.

Ideal yoga: Strength and empowerment classes to build muscle, stamina and emotional resilience.

Phase 3: Luteal phase (Inner Autumn/Waning Moon)

- Progesterone peaks, causing fatigue, bloating, sluggishness and lower serotonin (the happy hormone). May experience premenstrual symptoms such as tearfulness, irritability and mood swings.

Ideal yoga: Gentle restorative practices with forward folds or stretches to ease cramps. Slow breathing and introspective meditation can also be helpful.

Menstruation (Inner Winter/New Moon)

- This is your period. You may experience heavy or light bleeding, cramps or spotting.

Ideal yoga: Restorative yoga with forward folds or abdominal stretches to alleviate cramps. Slow breathing and meditation are encouraged.

PERIMENOPAUSE, MENOPAUSE AND POSTMENOPAUSE
Perimenopause
The time of transition from high oestrogen (Inner Summer) to high pro-gesterone (Inner Autumn). Like autumn weather, your moods and energy levels can be unpredictable. Hormone fluctuations can magnify existing symptoms.

- Key: Develop interoception (inner-body awareness) to understand your body's needs each day.
- Active days: Enjoy a more active yoga practice or physical exercise.
- Low energy days: Practise kindness and compassion towards your-self. Rest, reduce stress and choose gentler yoga practices such as yin yoga, restorative poses, breathing and meditation.

Menopause (Inner Winter)
Rest needs may increase, and joint/muscle aches, anxiety or insomnia may become more prominent. Hot flushes might persist.

Ideal yoga: Slow vinyasa yoga, somatic movements for joints and muscles, restorative yoga for sleep and practices to ease digestion (if bloating occurs).

Postmenopause (Second Spring)

This is a time of renewed energy and creativity. You may feel a resurgence similar to the follicular stage.

Ideal yoga: Consider a more active yoga practice and gradually rebuild strength and stamina. Strength classes, weight lifting, resistance training and impact exercises such as jogging or dancing might be suitable (although please consult a doctor before starting any new exercise programme).

Caution: Don't overdo it! Overstimulation can lead to burnout.

Low mood: Practise yoga classes designed to lift mood and combat lethargy if needed.

KEY TAKEAWAY

Listen to your body's unique needs throughout your cycle and during life stages. Yoga can be a powerful tool to support your wellbeing throughout these changes.

Creating a Menopause Yoga Home Practice

Understanding why you want to practise yoga and what you hope to gain helps you choose what to practise, when and how often. Yoga therapy uses SMART goals to help you create a daily practice you can sustain. SMART stands for:

- Specific. Clearly define what you want to achieve with your practice. This could be specific yoga poses, breathing exercises or meditations that target your symptoms, stage of menopause or desired time of day (e.g., morning stretches or evening relaxation techniques).
- Measurable. Set a way to track your progress. What do you hope to achieve through your practice? This could be a measurable outcome, such as reduced hot flushes, improved sleep or increased flexibility.
- Achievable. Be realistic about what you can accomplish with your time and limitations. Choose goals that fit your schedule, location and physical capabilities.
- Relevant. Make sure your goals align with your overall needs and desires. They should be something you truly want to achieve.
- Time-bound. Set a timeframe for achieving your goals. This could be a specific number of days you practise per week or the total duration of your yoga programme.

Remember, goals can be adjusted! Review your progress after a few weeks. See if your goals are still working for you or if they need to be tweaked to keep you motivated and on track.

CREATING A SMART DAILY PRACTICE AND STAYING MOTIVATED FOR SUCCESS

- Set SMART goals. Define clear, specific, measurable, achievable, relevant and time-bound goals to stay accountable. Share your intentions with a trusted friend or family member for added support.
- Track your progress. Maintain a journal to document your yoga practice, dietary choices and any changes you experience. Tracking symptoms, such as sleep patterns or hot flushes, can be insightful and motivating. For example, did eliminating afternoon coffee improve your sleep? Did reducing alcohol lessen night sweats? Does starting your day with a breathing technique, meditation and a positive intention (sankalpa) enhance your mood?
- Embrace flexibility. Review and adapt your plan as needed. If a particular breathing technique or yoga pose doesn't feel right, explore alternatives. Remember, this is your personal toolkit – so customize it for your needs.
- Keep it fresh. Positive habits are essential, but if your yoga practice becomes monotonous, explore new variations offered within this book.
- Share your journey. Discuss your learnings and insights from this book with friends. You might inspire them to make positive changes for their own wellbeing.

Use this blank template to set your own SMART goals.

Specific (What)	
Measurable (When/ duration)	

cont.

Achievable (How often)	
Relevant (Why)	
Time-bound (How long for/ commitment)	

COMMITMENT AND OPENNESS

As with any new endeavour, commitment and a willingness to explore are key to success. Whether you're new to yoga or this specific approach, Menopause Yoga offers a gentle and supportive practice.

BENEFITS OVER TIME AND STARTING NOW

With regular practice, the yoga, breathing and meditation techniques become easier. Begin now to have these tools readily available when you need them most.

Let's start together. Find your yoga mat or a comfortable place to sit, and let's begin.

Yoga basics: Breathwork

SEATED OCEAN BREATH (MODIFIED UJJAYI PRANAYAMA)

Ocean breath is a gentle breathing practice designed to release tension and promote relaxation.

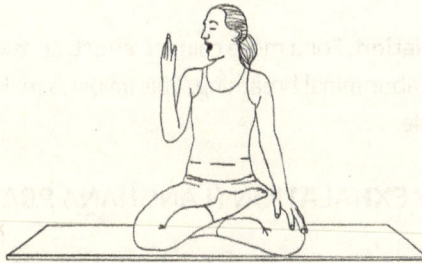

SEATED OCEAN BREATH (MODIFIED UJJAYI
PRANAYAMA), BEGINNER'S VERSION, WITH HAND

Benefits: This practice can stimulate the vagus nerve, which activates your parasympathetic nervous system (rest and digest response). The gentle sound can also soothe your nervous system, sending a message to relax. With practice, ocean breath can be your instant self-soothing tool that you can take with you anywhere and use any time you feel stressed or overwhelmed, and can cool hot flushes.

1. Inhale through the nose and allow your abdomen to relax as your breath fills your belly.
2. Subtle throat sound: As you exhale again through your nose, make a very quiet, barely audible, sound that resembles the sigh of the ocean. Imagine this sound gently stroking the back of your throat.
3. Focus on calm. Remember, this is not ujjayi (victorious) breath; it is the opposite function. Where ujjayi is heating, active, like the Sun, ocean breath through the mouth is like the cooling, calming, softer Moon.

ABDOMINAL BREATHING (ADHAM PRANAYAMA)

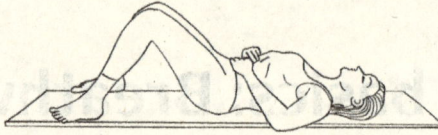

LYING DOWN (SUPINE) ABDOMINAL BREATHING
(ADHAM PRANAYAMA) WITH OCEAN BREATH

1. Start by lying down on your back.
2. Place one hand on your chest and the other on your belly.
3. Inhale slowly through your nose, feeling your belly expand as you inhale.
4. Exhale slowly and completely through your mouth or nose, feeling your belly contract as you exhale.

Ocean breath variation: For a more calming effect, consider incorporating ocean breath with abdominal breathing. This involves making a soft sighing sound on the exhale.

LONGER SLOW EXHALATION (LANGHANA PRANAYAMA)

Simple and effective, this is a great technique for beginners because it's gentle and avoids potentially increasing anxiety.

1. Inhale at your own pace. Breathe in for a comfortable count, for example 1, 2, 3.
2. Exhale longer. Exhale slowly and completely for a slightly longer count, for example 1, 2, 3, 4.
3. Gradually increase the exhale. As you feel more comfortable, gradually lengthen your exhale to the count of 5, 6, 7 or 8.

Listen to your body. If you feel anxious or short of breath at any time, stop, breathe naturally for a moment, and restart when you feel calm. You are in charge.

OXYTOCIN HUG

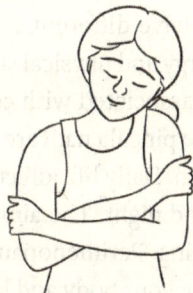

OXYTOCIN HUG

Benefits: You can experience the benefits of oxytocin, the feel-good hormone, even when physical touch is limited. This self-hug technique is meant to mimic the physical and emotional benefits of a hug. While it may not completely replace human contact, it can be a powerful tool for managing stress and promoting feelings of wellbeing, especially during times of social isolation. Here's a simple practice you can do anytime, anywhere:

1. Begin by rubbing the palms of your hands together briskly for 10 seconds. This generates warmth and stimulates nerve endings, preparing your body for the hug.
2. Take a deep breath in through your nose. As you inhale, open your arms wide as if you're about to embrace someone you love dearly. Imagine their presence and the warmth of their touch.
3. As you slowly exhale through your mouth, gently hug yourself. Wrap your arms around your torso and hold for a comfortable moment.
4. Maintain your self-hug while slowly stroking your upper arms with your hands. Imagine waves of relaxation flowing down your body with each stroke. Breathe deeply and evenly throughout this step.
5. While holding the self-hug and stroking your arms, focus on the feeling of comfort and security. Imagine the oxytocin releasing and promoting feelings of relaxation and connection, even in the absence of physical contact with another person.

There is no set duration for this practice. Perform the self-hug for as long as it feels beneficial. You can repeat this exercise throughout the day whenever you feel stressed or isolated.

BALANCING BREATHING TECHNIQUES

In Traditional Chinese Medicine (TCM) and Indian Ayurveda health systems, it is believed we have different energies flowing through us, affecting our thoughts, energy and physical state. In TCM, yin and the ida nadi (energy channel) are associated with cool, calm, reflective energy, like the Moon. Yang and the pingala nadi are associated with heat, active dynamic energy, like the Sun. Daily life affects the balance of these energies, which fluctuate day and night. The aim is to stay balanced on both sides for health and wellbeing. Perimenopause to menopause is a major hormone upheaval affecting your body and brain that may cause a sense of imbalance in mind, body and emotions. These breathing techniques cannot replace the hormones that are naturally changing, but they may help ease some of your symptoms to give you a sense of balance (sattva).

TIPS

- Be patient with yourself. It takes practice to master these techniques.
- If one technique doesn't work for you, try another.
- There is no 'one size fits all' approach. Find what works best for you and put it in your 'MY toolkit'. The Toolkit is part of 'Creating a Menopause Yoga Home Practice' that meets the individual person's needs.

BALANCING BREATH (ANULOMA PRANAYAMA)

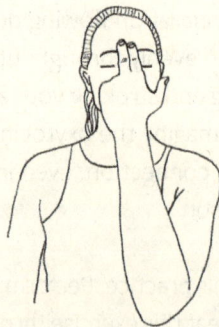

BALANCING BREATH (ANULOMA PRANAYAMA)

Benefits: This simple technique is a good way to check in with your energy and breathing – and it is good for beginners to practise breath control (pranayama).

1. Rest your 1st and 2nd fingers on your forehead or between your eyebrows for a sense of mental calm.
2. Lightly rest your thumb on one nostril and your ring (3rd) finger on the other nostril.
3. Inhale through both nostrils, pause for a second and close your right nostril. Then breathe out of your left nostril.
4. Inhale through both nostrils, pause for a second, then close your left nostril and only breathe out of your right nostril.
5. Breathe in through both nostrils, pause, then close your right nostril and only breathe out of your left nostril.
6. Repeat 3 rounds of 10 breaths (or start with 5 rounds of breath if you are a beginner) and then relax your hands, breathe naturally, and notice if you are breathing more through one nostril. This is natural and changes through the day and night, but if you feel very one-sided, you can balance out your breath and energy by using alternate nostril breath, left nostril breathing, right nostril breathing.

ALTERNATE NOSTRIL BREATHING (NADI SHODHANA)

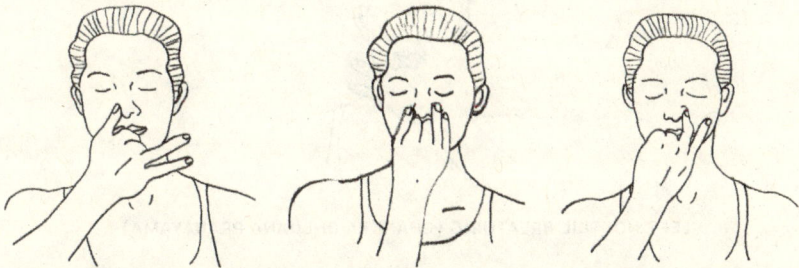

ALTERNATIVE NOSTRIL BREATHING (ANULOMA VILLOMA OR NADI SHODHANA)

1. Get comfortable. Sit upright in a chair with a straight spine.
2. Use your thumb to gently close your right nostril. Inhale through your left nostril, pause, close your left nostril, open your right nostril.

3. Exhale through your right nostril. Pause, close your right nostril, open your left nostril. Exhale through your left nostril.
4. Repeat the practice, alternating nostrils for 5–10 rounds. End with an exhalation out of your left nostril. Relax your hand and breathe naturally. Observe how you feel.

Challenge: Pause for a few seconds longer at the top of your inhalation (antara kumbhaka, retention of breath) and then at the bottom of your exhalation (bahir kumbhaka, holding the exhalation).

Please note: Avoid breath retention if you have anxiety or panic attacks, or issues with blood pressure, eyes or ears.

Remember: If you feel anxious at any time, *stop* this breathing practice and breathe naturally. You can try 'Balancing breath (anuloma pranayama), beginner's version, with both nostrils'.

LEFT NOSTRIL BREATHING (CHANDRA BHEDANA PRANAYAMA)

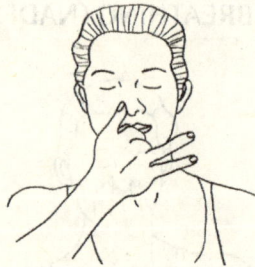

LEFT NOSTRIL BREATHING (CHANDRA BHEDANA PRANAYAMA)

Benefits: This cooling, calming left nostril breathing is associated with ida nadi, the cooling, calming side of your brain and body, so it may help reduce feelings of heat and anger associated with hot flushes and menopause rage. The left nostril is linked to the cool calmness of the Moon. Breathe in and out only through your left nostril.

1. Sit comfortably, upright in a chair, with a straight spine.
2. Raise the hand that is most comfortable for you and touch your thumb lightly on your right nostril and your ring (3rd) finger on the left nostril. You can either rest your middle two fingers on your forehead for a sense of mental calm, or simply tuck them out of the way, along with your little (4th) finger. Close your eyes, if this is comfortable for you, or look down to the ground.
3. Close your right nostril using your thumb. Inhale through the left nostril. Pause for 1–2 seconds at the top of your inhalation. Exhale through your left nostril.
4. Repeat, inhaling and exhaling only through your left nostril, for 3 x 10 rounds of breath – or as many as feels comfortable.
5. Relax both hands and breathe naturally. Observe your breathing and how you feel.

RIGHT NOSTRIL BREATHING (SURYA BHEDANA PRANAYAMA)

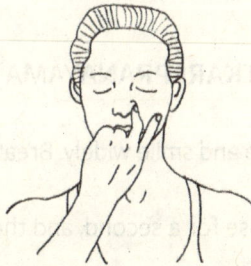

RIGHT NOSTRIL BREATHING (SURYA BHEDANA PRANAYAMA)

This is the same practice as left nostril breathing, but change hands and breathe in and out only through your right nostril. The right nostril is linked to pingala nadi and the active, heating side of your brain and body, so right nostril breathing may feel more energizing and heating if you feel lethargic or experience cold chills.

113

COOLING BREATH TECHNIQUES

Here are three cooling breath techniques to help manage hot flushes.

STRAW BREATH (KAKI PRANAYAMA)

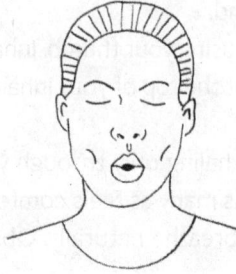

STRAW BREATH (KAKI PRANAYAMA)

1. Suck in the air as you inhale through pursed lips, as if using a straw. Breathe in slowly through your pursed lips.
2. Close your mouth, pause for a second, and then exhale slowly through your nose.

SMILING BREATH (SITKARI PRANAYAMA)

1. Open your mouth wide and smile widely. Breathe in slowly through the sides of your mouth.
2. Close your mouth, pause for a second, and then exhale slowly through your nose.

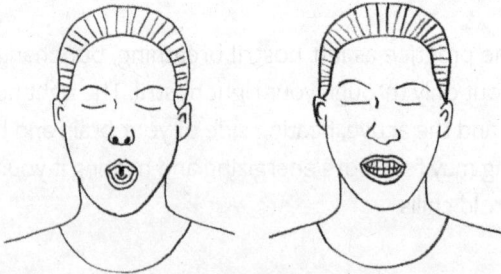

COOLING BREATH (SITALI AND SITKARI PRANAYAMA)

COOLING (OR FUNNEL) BREATH (SITALI PRANAYAMA), WITH CURLED TONGUE

1. Curl the sides of your tongue and suck in air through the funnel shape.
2. Close your mouth, pause for a second, and then exhale slowly through your nose.

Tips: The open mouth cools the air as you inhale due to the evaporation of saliva. The long exhale through the nose calms the mind. The longer the exhale, the calmer you'll feel.

Start with exaggerated mouth positions as you learn the techniques, and then gradually soften your mouth and lips so that you can practise these breathing tools in a public place, without people noticing.

HOT FLUSH WAVE, WITH OCEAN BREATH

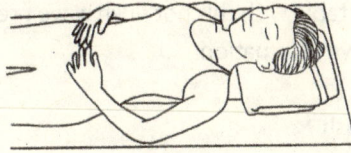

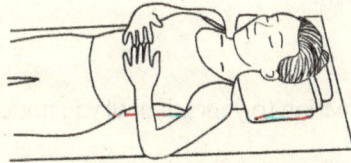

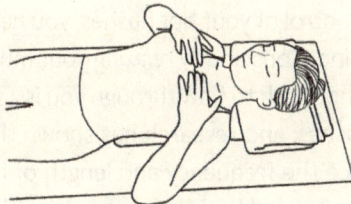

HOT FLUSH WAVE, WITH OCEAN BREATH

1. Place your hands on your abdomen and breathe into the space beneath your hands to feel your navel rise as you inhale and soften and relax as

you exhale. Breathe in through your nose, and exhale slowly out of your mouth with the calming sound of your ocean breath.

2. Place your hands on your lower ribs. Inhale into the space beneath your hands, pause for a second, and exhale out of your mouth as you soften the ribs, making the ocean breath sound.

3. Place your hands on your chest. Inhale through your nose as you breathe into the space beneath your fingers. Pause for a second, then exhale out of your mouth with ocean breath sound.

4. Now imagine a hot flush starting in your abdomen. You can choose to visualize the hot flush as a colour or a warm feeling. As you inhale, allow that colour or warmth to rise up from your abdomen to your ribs, and then up to your chest and neck – then open your mouth and exhale, letting the heat release with ocean breath sound.

5. Repeat this style of breathing, releasing the heat out of your mouth each time and relaxing your jaw. This sounds like a soft, cooling wave and feels like a sigh of relief as you let it go.

When you are comfortable with this hot flush wave breathing and visualization, add in this positive affirmation:

This is just a hot flush
It will not last
I let it flow through me
The heat will pass.

Say this rhyming affirmation to yourself until you notice yourself becoming cooler and calmer.

Remember: To take control of your hot flushes, you need to both cool your body and calm your mind. Consciously *relaxing* your muscles, your body, and *choosing* to allow the hot flush to flow through you is a way to feel in control of your erratic hot flushes, and research has shown this 'paced breathing' style will help to reduce the frequency and length of hot flushes in future. You are training your mind and body to respond calmly to the heat instead of triggering a stress response.

SOOTHING MENOPAUSE RAGE

Menopause rage is a physical and psychological sense of anger that appears to surge from 0 to 100 in seconds. In that moment, you may feel 100 per cent justified in your rage about someone or something. Afterwards, give yourself some loving kindness – you were just having a human emotion. Practise these techniques when you are feeling good so that you can use them when you are feeling overwhelmed with irritability. (See 'MY class for menorage and irritability'.)

Let's begin with an exaggerated technique called lion's breath. You are literally going to let out all your pent-up anger or irritability with a roar and your most frightening facial expression. Practising this looking in the mirror may make you laugh, and laughter is a quick fix to feeling better.

LION'S BREATH (SIMHASANA PRANAYAMA)

1. Inhale through your nose deeply, and then open your mouth, tongue down towards your chin, and open your eyes wide as you breathe out, making a roaring sound like a lion.
2. Repeat for 4–8 breaths. This is releasing your pent-up unexpressed rage and irritability in a way that is not directed at others or yourself. Look in the mirror when you do this – it may make you smile at yourself. Remember, you are just having a human emotion; it is neither good nor bad.
3. Afterwards, give yourself an oxytocin hug and embrace yourself with compassion. Start by positively reframing your feelings. Instead of feeling guilty for being angry (you are just having a human emotion) or being consumed by a sense of feeling 100 per cent justified in your rage, focus instead on soothing yourself with kindness and compassion.

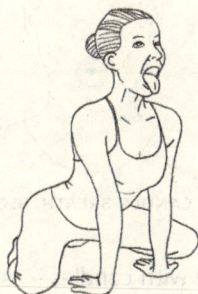

LION'S BREATH (SIMHASANA PRANAYAMA)

LETTING OFF STEAM (HISSING BREATH)

Benefits: This breathing technique helps you let off steam, releasing rising tension. It sounds like a snake, or the steam escaping from a pressure cooker.

1. Inhale through your nose, pause, and smile, with your teeth showing.
2. Exhale out of your mouth making a hissing 'sssss' sound, with your tongue behind your teeth.
3. Repeat 3 x 10 rounds of breaths.

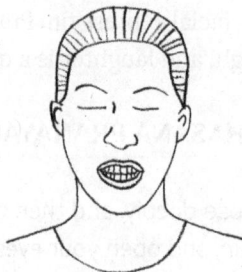

HISSING BREATH

Tip: Start with a wide smile and a strong, loud hissing sound to release pressure, and then relax your mouth into a gentle smile and exhale with a softer sound, like the air escaping from a slow bicycle puncture.

BLOWING BIRTHDAY CANDLE BREATH

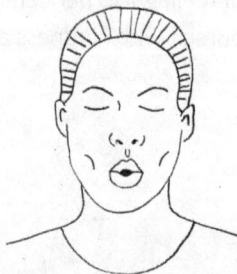

BLOWING BIRTHDAY CANDLE BREATH, BLOWING THE AIR OUT

1. Visualize a birthday cake with candles – as many as your age. This is a celebration of you and the life you have lived so far, so you can make it the most delicious cake you like.

2. Inhale through your nose to take a deep breath, and then exhale to slowly blow out some of the candles – but not all at once.
3. Then, exhale more slowly and softly – there are fewer candles to blow out. Blow as softly and as long as you can until the final flame is blown out.
4. Repeat for 10 breaths.

Tip: At the start, you'll want to take a deep breath and blow strongly – there may be a lot of candles.

BREATHWORK FOR CALMING ANXIETY AND OVERWHELM

Feeling anxious or overwhelmed? Here are a few breathwork techniques you can try to manage those feelings and find your centre.

BOX BREATHING (4-2-4-2)

1. Start with lying down (supine) abdominal breathing (adham pranayama).
2. Breathe in slowly through your nose for a count of four.
3. Briefly hold your breath after the inhale for a count of two.
4. Exhale slowly and completely through your mouth or nose for a count of four.
5. Briefly hold your breath after the exhale for a count of two.
6. Repeat this cycle for 10 rounds, or until you feel calmer.

Modify as needed: If holding your breath for two counts feels uncomfortable, shorten the hold to one count, until you build experience.

Challenge: Practise the same techniques with a breath count ratio of 4-4-4-4.

GROUNDING BREATH

1. Connect to the earth. Stand with your feet wider than hip distance apart, parallel, and knees slightly bent. Maintain an upright spine and allow your tailbone to drop naturally towards the ground.
2. Inhale through your nose, raise your arms out to the sides and overhead. Briefly hold at the top of the inhale.

3. Turn your palms down, softening your hands.
4. Exhale out of your mouth, making a soft 'haaaa' ocean sound, slowly bend your knees and press your hands down through the centre of your body. Imagine your hands pressing down with resistance, like a French coffee press.
5. Repeat this cycle for 10 rounds.

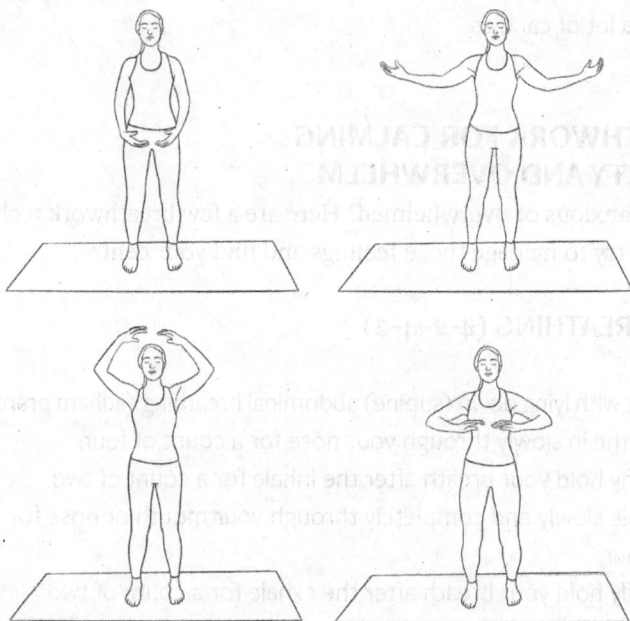

GROUNDING BREATH, PARTS 1–4

STRAP BREATH

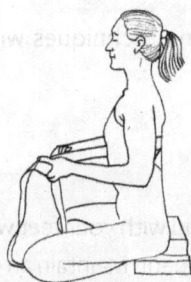

SEATED STRAP BREATHING

Part 1

1. Place a yoga belt or strap around the back of your rib cage, positioned at the bottom of your shoulder blades (not in the armpits). Gently hug your elbows into the rib cage and reach your hands forward holding the strap, so that your arms are at a right angle. Avoid hunching your shoulders.
2. Wrap the strap around your hands and hold lightly. The ribs should be able to move freely with your breath.
3. Close your eyes, or look to the floor, and inhale deeply into the back of your rib cage. Exhale, and relax your ribs.
4. Repeat 10 times, following the gentle expansion and contraction.

Part 2

1. Cross the strap in front of your chest and hold it lightly in opposite hands. You should be able to breathe easily.
2. Focus on breathing into the sides of your rib cage, feeling the strap and your lungs expand and contract. You are moving your muscles with the power of your breath.

Part 3

1. Release the strap and place your hands at the heart centre of your chest.
2. Breathe into your hands, feeling your ribs expand forward and back.

Visualization: Imagine your heart is expanding with every inhalation and contracting on every exhalation. Think of someone who brings you joy or happiness, or someone who is in need of kindness and having their spirits lifted. As you inhale, feel your heart expand, and send love, healing and kindness to whoever needs it. As you exhale, allow that compassion to return to your heart, nourishing you. You can visualize the heart as a colour or a light or a warmth that grows with every inhalation, filling your chest. Repeat 10 times and then relax and notice how you feel.

BREATHWORK TO LIFT LOW MOOD AND LETHARGY, AND CLEAR BRAIN FOG AND FATIGUE

Feeling low or sluggish? These breathwork techniques can help lift your spirits and energize your body.

MODIFIED BELLOWS BREATH (BHASTRIKA PRANAYAMA) AND GENTLE SKULL SHINING BREATH (KAPALABHATI PRANAYAMA)

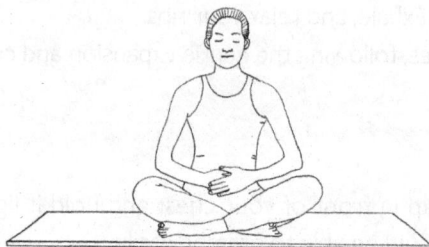

MODIFIED BELLOWS BREATH (SLOW KAPALABHATI BREATHING)

Benefits: This modified approach aims to create an uplifting and inspiring effect on your mind and body.

1. Start in a comfortable seated position with your hands resting lightly on your abdomen. Allow your abdomen to soften and relax into the palms of your hands as you breathe deeply.
2. Begin a slow bellows breath by inhaling through your nose, relaxing your abdomen into the palms of your hands, and then sharply exhale as if you were sneezing, pulling your abdomen in towards your spine.
3. Repeat 10 rounds of breathing slowly, and then relax and breathe normally for 1–2 breaths.
4. Repeat another 2 x 10 rounds, breathing slowly and resting in between, to check how you feel.

Caution: If at any time you feel dizzy or anxious, slow down your breathing pace or *stop* this practice. Return to your own natural breathing.

For slow and controlled breathing: Breathe slowly and gently, avoiding any forceful or aggressive movements.

BREATH OF JOY

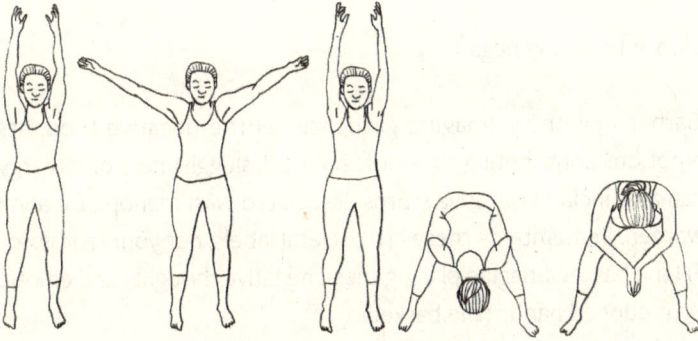

BREATH OF JOY, STANDING

1. Inhale, raise your arms up. Exhale, lower your arms. Inhale, open your arms out to the side, exhale, lower your arms. Inhale, raise your arms above your head, exhale out of our mouth, making a 'haaaa' sound as you bend your knees and fold forward, sweeping your arms behind you.

2. Inhale as you bend your knees and stand upright with a straight spine, arms raised over your head. Repeat for 10 rounds.

3. If you have high or low blood pressure, regular hot flushes or migraines, keep your head level with your heart. Rest your elbows on your thighs with a straight spine as you fold forward.

4. Everyone else can bend their knees and allow their back to relax as they fold forward.

FOUNTAIN BREATH

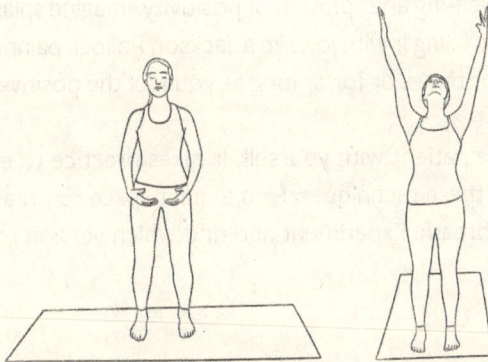

GROUNDING BREATH, PART 1 AND FOUNTAIN BREATH, PART 2, WITH ARMS RAISED

1. Place your hands on your abdomen, just below your navel, with palms facing up. Gently close your eyes if comfortable.

Version 1: Releasing negativity

1. Gather negativity. Imagine gathering all the negative thoughts and emotions contributing to your low mood, sluggishness or lethargy. You can also include negative words associated with menopause and older women. Remember – these are societal labels, not your truths.
2. Fill the basket. Imagine placing these negative thoughts and emotions in your cupped hands (the basket).
3. Inhale and release. As you inhale, bring your hands to your chest and pause. Then, turn your palms upwards, releasing your arms and hands towards the sky while straightening your legs. Exhale and release all those negative words, thoughts and emotions. Repeat this process four times, or until you feel lighter and more positive.

Version 2: Embracing positivity

1. Gather positivity. Imagine collecting all the positive thoughts about yourself, your life, what brings you joy and your favourite colours. You can also add fireworks, sparkles and positive words about your menopause journey. Own these positive descriptions.
2. Fill the basket. Place these positive thoughts and emotions in your cupped hands (the basket).
3. Inhale and expand. As you inhale, bring your hands up to your heart and pause. Then, turn your palms upwards and exhale, straightening your legs, as if releasing an explosion of positivity. Imagine splashing the walls of the room, filling it with joy, like a Jackson Pollock painting. Repeat this process four times, or for as long as you feel the positive effects.

Remember: Be patient with yourself. It takes practice to experience the full benefits of these techniques. Find a quiet space to breathe freely, and focus on your breath. Experiment and find which version resonates most with you.

By incorporating these breathwork techniques into your routine, you can combat low mood and lethargy, replacing them with a renewed sense of energy and positivity. Watch and practice these breathing technique videos.

TUPLER BREATHING OR STAR BREATH

Tupler exercises are seated on the mat. The Tupler Technique® can specifically help people with diastasis recti (the gap between your abdominal muscles) that often occurs after pregnancy or surgery. This technique helps women to engage their rectus abdominis muscles, which may separate as a result of pregnancy or a sedentary lifestyle.

1. Seated: Sit upright with feet flat on the floor, or lie on your back with your knees bent and the soles of your feet on the floor.
2. Place one hand above your navel and one hand below. Visualize a star radiating horizontally from your navel out to the sides of your waist and diagonally across your abdomen, connecting the left lower ribs to the right hip bone and the right lower ribs to the left hip bone (like a union jack flag).
3. Inhale as you allow your belly to soften, exhale and squeeze from these six points of the star into the centre of your navel, and then draw this point back towards your spine.
4. Hold here for 2–4 counts. Inhale as you relax your belly.
5. Repeat for 10 rounds.

Challenge: As you gain muscle control, challenge yourself to hold in for longer. Then relax and notice how you feel. Repeat this longer hold for 1 round several times a day.

Yoga basics: Mudras, mantras and meditation for menopause

This section explores how incorporating mudras (hand gestures), mantras (chants) and meditation into your yoga practice can help manage menopausal symptoms and cultivate a sense of acceptance.

WHAT ARE MUDRAS?

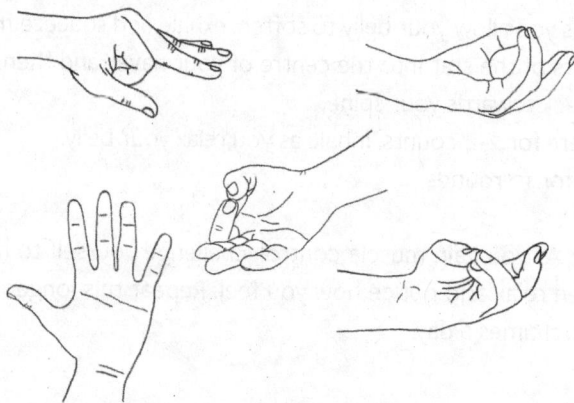

MIXED HAND MUDRA

Mudras are symbolic hand gestures used in yoga and meditation to channel energy flow (prana) within the body. Regularly practising mudras with meditation can improve mental clarity and emotional wellbeing. Here are some mudras that can be incorporated into your Menopause Yoga practice.

WOMB-SPACE GESTURE (YONI MUDRA)

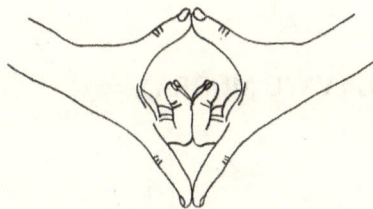

WOMB-SPACE GESTURE (YONI MUDRA)

In Ayurveda, this traditional mudra is said to benefit women experiencing hormonal imbalances related to menopause. I prefer women regularly placing the palms of their hands on their abdomen and allowing the warmth to bring comfort and connection to a part of their body that may feel sore, bloated and associated with menstrual pain or surgery.

1. Create a heart shape by touching both thumbs and 1st fingers together.
2. Place one over your heart and one hand on your 'womb space'.
3. Breathe deeply into both.
4. Send some loving kindness from your heart to your womb space.

GESTURE OF WISDOM (JNANA MUDRA)

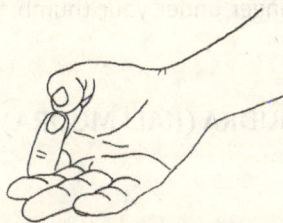

GESTURE OF WISDOM (JNANA MUDRA)

This mudra promotes a sense of wisdom and knowledge. It is also known as chin mudra, and can be practised for mental clarity if the palm of the hand is turned upwards.

1. Touch the tip of your index (1st) finger to the tip of your thumb, forming a circle. Keep the remaining three fingers extended. Rest the backs of your hands on your thighs or knees, with palms facing up.

2. This mudra can be practised in any yoga pose, but it's most commonly used in seated positions, like easy pose (sukhasana) or lotus pose (padmasana).

VATA BALANCING (VAYU MUDRA)

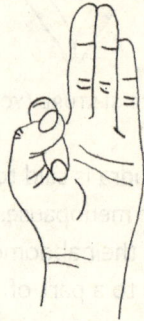

VATA BALANCING (VAYU MUDRA)

This mudra helps to reduce stress, anxiety, bloating, flatulence and joint pain associated with vata dosha imbalances.

1. Sit comfortably on the mat or chair (it helps to lean your spine against an upturned bolster) and position your hands, either with palms facing down on the legs, to invite a sense of grounding, or folding the knuckle of your index (1st) finger under your thumb, for a sense of calm and connection.

LIGHTNING BOLT MUDRA (KALI MUDRA)

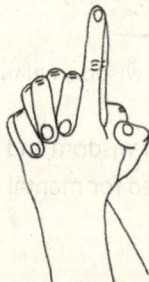

LIGHTNING BOLT MUDRA (KALI MUDRA)

I love the idea of Goddess Kali, the fierce protector and destroyer who is respected and revered in Indian classical culture. I think we can all benefit from channelling a bit of Goddess Kali as we go through our menopause, learning to challenge social stereotypes of women in menopause, and using her lightning bolt to cut through discrimination.

1. Interlace the fingers of both hands and cross your thumbs.
2. Point your index (1st) fingers up together to create an arrow or lightning bolt.
3. Lift your hands in the lightning bolt as you inhale, releasing the arms on your exhale.

GODDESS HAKINI MUDRA

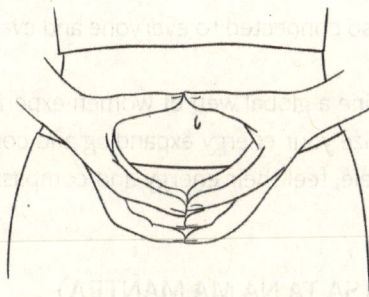

GODDESS HAKINI MUDRA

This mudra brings everything into the right place and can help you to feel balanced.

1. Touch the thumb and fingertips of your left hand to the thumb and fingertips of your right hand.
2. Place your hands in front of your navel.
3. Imagine you are holding a golden ball of energy in between your hands.
4. After 10 breaths, touch the palms of both hands on your abdomen and imagine this golden ball of energy nourishing you.

COMBINING MUDRAS WITH MANTRAS

'I AM THAT' (SO-HAM MANTRA)

Benefits: This visualization can help alleviate feelings of isolation and remind you that you're not alone in this journey through menopause.

1. Start with your hands in vata balancing (vayu mudra) for a sense of calm and connection that can feel grounding.
2. Repeat the mantra 'so' as you inhale' and 'ham/hum' as you exhale. Repeat 10 times, and then repeat the mantra silently in your mind.

Focus on the sense of expansion in your body as you inhale and the soft contraction as you exhale. This mantra reminds us that we are both an individual person and also connected to everyone and everything.

Visualization: Imagine a global web of women experiencing menopause. As you inhale, visualize your energy expanding and connecting with these women. As you exhale, feel their energy and compassion returning back to you.

'MY TRUE SELF' (SA TA NA MA MANTRA)

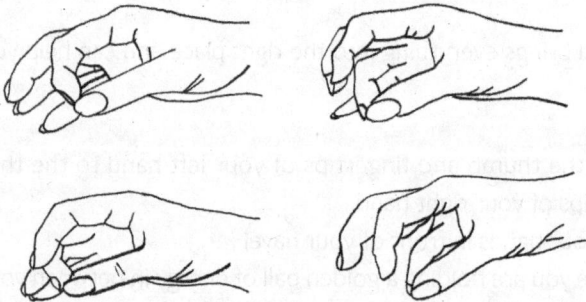

'MY TRUE SELF' (SA TA NA MA MANTRA)

I have modified this practice to be much slower than the traditional cleansing (kriya) used in kundalini yoga. The focus of this practice is on your slow exhalation as you change your thumb and finger positions, with your eyes closed. The meaning of the mantra sounds 'sa, ta, na, ma' reminds us of the natural changes in the stages of life and Nature's cyclical seasons. It invites us to accept the life changes from perimenopause (Autumn) to menopause (Winter), so that we can reemerge transformed into postmenopause (Second Spring).

Sanskrit meaning:

- *Sa:* Birth, beginning and the totality of the cosmos.
- *Ta:* Life, existence and creativity.
- *Na:* Death and transformation.
- *Ma:* Rebirth, regeneration and experiencing the joy of the Infinite.

If the concept of reincarnation does not resonate with you, replace this with the 'Seasons of Nature: Spring, Summer, Autumn, Winter, Second Spring'.

1. Inhale through your nose with both palms of your hands open. Exhale out of your mouth saying the sound 'saaaa' as you touch your thumb to your 1st finger.
2. Inhale through your nose. Exhale out of your mouth saying the sound 'taaaa' and touch your thumb to your 2nd finger.
3. Inhale through your nose. Exhale saying 'naaaa' as you touch your thumb to your 3rd finger.
4. Inhale through your nose. Exhale saying 'maaaa' and touch your thumb to your little finger.
5. Repeat this cycle for two rounds saying the sounds like a singing chant, then two rounds whispering and then two rounds silently in your mind. Sit quietly and observe your breathing, your thoughts (are they quiet or busy?) and your emotions.

Tip: This has many mind-calming purposes, but I use this slow, modified version for soothing menopause rage because it distracts the mind away from irritable thoughts. (See 'MY class for menorage and irritability'.)

YOGA NIDRA

Yoga nidra is the practice of conscious sleep where the body is completely relaxed but the mind is still conscious. Rooted in ancient India, it is also known as 'yogic sleep'. The benefits of yoga nidra include overcoming stress, insomnia and fatigue.

Here are some examples of yoga nidra that you may like to record on your phone and listen to while you are relaxing in the restorative poses or a simple abdominal breathing practice.

CALM POND YOGA NIDRA

1. Close your eyes and breathe deeply.
2. Imagine a peaceful pond surrounded by reeds. Notice the water's surface – is it calm or rippled?
3. A single leaf floats down and gently lands. As you breathe deeply, visualize the leaf slowly sinking, taking your stress with it.
4. Hold this image for eight breaths, feeling tranquillity wash over you.
5. Then, see the leaf effortlessly rise back to the surface. Breathe deeply, feeling calm.
6. When you are ready, gently open your eyes, carrying this peace with you.

Remember: There's no right or wrong way to practise this. The key is to find what feels comfortable and beneficial for you.

YOGA NIDRA FOR GROUNDING AND CALMING ANXIETY

Use your sense of touch:

1. Find a comfortable seated position, perhaps sitting in a chair with your feet flat on the floor, or with a wall behind you for support.
2. Rest the palms of your hands on your knees or thighs.
3. Focus on your feet – spread your toes wide and open the soles of your feet into the ground beneath you. Imagine your feet are the roots of a tree reaching down into the earth beneath you. Notice if these roots make you feel steady, stable, grounded. Say to yourself, 'I am grounded, I am anchored, I am safe.'
4. As you gently root down through your feet, do you notice a subtle lift and lengthening along your spine all the way up to your neck? How does this feel?

Use your sense of sight:

1. Close your eyes, then open them wide.
2. Find two to three objects to focus your gaze on and look at them as if you are seeing them for the first time. What do you notice about the colour, shape, texture of each? Where does the light shine on them? Can you name each of these observations? For instance: sky, clouds, sunlight, deep blue, grey, white, yellow. Flowerpot, roses, pink and yellow, petals, soft, velvet.

Use your sense of smell:

1. Close your eyes and breathe in deeply, allowing your nostrils to open wide to receive the air.
2. Notice if there are any aromas in the air. If there are, can you label them? Avoid getting drawn into a dialogue about them. Just name each one and let them go.

Use your sense of movement:

1. As you breathe deeply, soften your abdomen so that as you inhale the belly gently rises, and as you exhale, it softens back down.
2. Notice what happens when you relax your lower jaw and soften all the muscles on your face. Does your belly rise and fall more softly? Is it easier to breathe more deeply?
3. Continue this belly breath, but try extending the exhalation for an extra second or two. Avoid forcing your breath, just let it expand naturally. Observe how the breath is creating movement within your body.
4. Continue breathing like this for 8–10 more rounds before completing the practice. Observe how you feel, or move on to the next stage, deeper breath awareness (viloma pranayama).

Deeper breath awareness (viloma pranayama), 3-part breath

1. Allow the breath to slowly drain out naturally. After a few rounds, extend the inhalation into the upper chest at the collar bones, feeling the belly, front and sides of the rib cage expand to make space for the lungs.
2. Extend the exhalation even by one or two seconds, which will slow the heart rate down slightly and calm the nervous system.
3. Continue for 8–10 more rounds, counting quietly to yourself.

Self-soothing affirmation: On your exhalations, repeat these words: 'I am safe, I am loved, I am cared for, I am supported by Mother Earth beneath me.'

Body scan and relaxation (savasana)

1. Find a comfortable lying position, either with feet flat, legs long or raised on a chair, and use props where necessary to ensure that you are not distracted by cold or heat or physical discomfort.
2. Slowly scan your body, inviting each part to yield into the ground beneath you and become heavy.
3. When you've completed the full body scan, drop into relaxation for a minimum of 5–15 minutes.
4. Return to an upright seated position of your choice and take a few moments to observe how you are feeling.
5. Place one hand at the centre of your chest and the other hand on top.
6. Notice your heartbeat and the steady rise and fall of your chest as you breathe.
7. Imagine your heart was gently expanding towards the palms of your hands on the inhalation and softening back inwards on the exhalation. Imagine your heart as a colour, shape or light that gently expands like the petals of a lotus flower as you inhale. It feels as if your heart is growing bigger with every round of breath.

Loving kindness

1. As you inhale, feel your heart grow and send loving kindness to another person or people.
2. As you exhale, allow that loving kindness to bathe you in its warmth.

MIND MEETS THE BREATH MEDITATION

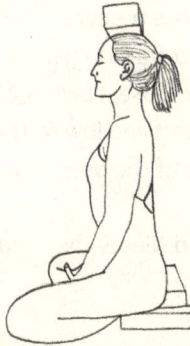

MIND MEETS THE BREATH

1. Sit comfortably with your spine upright and your abdomen relaxed so that you can breathe easily. Sitting against a wall or on blocks, or a straight-backed chair can support your back.
2. Balance a cork brick on the crown of your head (a wooden brick is too heavy and may slip; a foam block is too light). Alternatively, place a low-weight eye pillow on the crown of your head. This is a marma point (an Ayurvedic acupressure point) and the gentle pressure can feel calming.
3. Rest your hands on your legs with palms down, which feels grounding. Close your eyes if you feel comfortable doing so.
4. Focus on your breath, breathing slowly and steadily so that your inhalation and exhalation are of equal length. The aim is to slow your breath down but without holding your breath. This is not a breath retention (khumbhaka) exercise. Stay here for 3–5 minutes and count how many rounds of breath you took in this time.
5. To come out of the pose, slowly raise one hand towards your head, moving in slow motion – fast movement will disturb your nervous system. Touch the brick or eye bag and lift it off your head, pausing for a few breaths to observe how this feels. Then slowly lower the brick or eye bag from your head, keeping your eyes closed, and rest it on the ground, making no sound as it touches the floor.

6. Rest both hands on your legs and sit quietly for a few minutes. Notice if the mental activity in your mind has slowed down or if you feel calmer and more at peace. This pose prepares us for a deeper meditation practice, so you may choose to stay longer.

7. When you come out of this pose, slowly flutter your eyes open, keeping your gaze soft and low so that you slowly receive the light and sight of the outside world.

Watch and practice this Mind Meets the Breath meditation to help calm anxiety.

THIRD EYE SEATED MEDITATION

1. Sit comfortably upright in a chair, with your feet touching the floor for a sense of grounding.

2. Close your eyes and breathe slowly in and out of your nose.

3. Take your inner gaze to the place slightly above and between your eyebrows. This is your third eye (dristi), which simply means a place to focus your attention. Draw your gaze inwards to the centre of your head, which may feel as if you are 'cross-eyed'. Stay here for several minutes, or as long as your attention will allow. Then relax your eyes and notice how you feel.

4. To exit, either cover your eyes with your hands or blink your eyes open and allow them to adjust to the light.

LOVING-KINDNESS MEDITATION (METTA BHAVANA)

This simple loving-kindness meditation is a method of developing compassion. It comes from the Buddhist tradition, but it can be adapted and practised by anyone, regardless of religious affiliation; it is essentially about cultivating love. At the heart of this meditation is self-acceptance. Once we take care of ourselves, we have a deeper well from which to draw compassion for others.

May I be filled with loving kindness, may I be peaceful and at ease.
May she be filled with loving kindness, may she be peaceful and at ease.

May they be filled with loving kindness, may they be peaceful and at ease. May we all be filled with loving kindness; may we all be peaceful and at ease.

METTA MEDITATION, LEVEL 2

When you are comfortable with the meditation techniques, you may want to practice the level 2 version of the meta meditation. This helps release negative emotions such as fear and pain. Please watch and listen to the video first, and decide if this is a suitable practice for you.

If you are feeling overwhelmed, listen to this calming Guided Visualisation for Sense Withdrawl plus some other recorded meditations and yoga nidras.

Yoga basics: Props and modifications for menopause

Prop *your* body, not the pose.

Props support your body physically and emotionally; they can enhance your practice and keep you warm, and they can make the poses and meditation more comfortable.

Essential props:

- Yoga mat: provides cushioning and prevents slipping.

Optional but helpful props:

- Bolster: a firm, cylindrical cushion for support in restorative poses.
- Weighted eye bag: applies gentle pressure on your eyes or forehead for deep relaxation.
- Yoga bricks (x2): brick-shaped props for added height or support in poses.
- Strap/belt: increases your reach and flexibility in certain poses.
- Blankets: for warmth and body support in restorative poses and easing joint discomfort.

You can also use everyday household items as substitutes:

- Cushions (firm) can replace a bolster.
- A small bag filled with rice or beans can be a weighted sandbag alternative.

- Large books can act as yoga blocks.
- A scarf or belt can be used as a yoga strap.
- A chair.

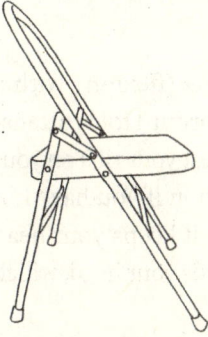

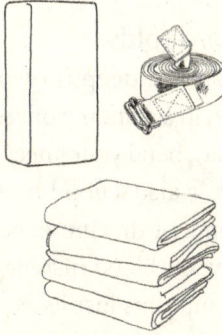

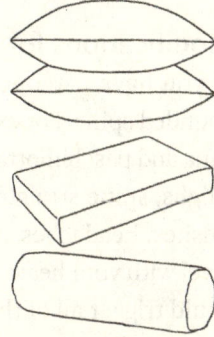

PROPS: CHAIR   PROPS: BLOCK, BLANKETS, BELTS   PROPS: CUSHIONS, BLOCK, BOLSTER

USING PROPS FOR MODIFICATIONS

Menopause brings a wave of physical and emotional changes, which can be overwhelming. Yoga can be a powerful tool to navigate this transition, but a one-size-fits-all approach won't work. You may have seen Lycra-clad yoga teachers performing pretzel poses or gravity-defying balances. This is not Menopause Yoga. My practice invites you to adapt your practice to your unique individual needs and embrace the journey of self-discovery. Use props, including cushions, blankets, belt, blocks, bolsters, etc. It's not a sign of weakness; it's a radical act of self-care.

Adaptability extends beyond postures. You can tailor your breathing techniques, hand positions (mudras), mantras (repeated sounds or words) and affirmations. For instance, two rapid breathing techniques – called bellows breath (slow kapalabhati breathing) and skull shining breath (kapalabhati pranayama) – are traditionally used in yoga as cleansing (kriya) for mental clarity. However, in perimenopause, this style of breathing could trigger a panic or anxiety attack in people with a history of these conditions. So, in Menopause Yoga, and as seen in 'Yoga basics: Breathwork', we modify this breathing technique by slowing down the pace, focusing on a long exhale to calm your nervous system, while gently clearing your brain fog. It can effectively feel like you've blown away the cobwebs and can now think clearly afterwards. Try it for yourself and see.

During the menopause we benefit from modifications. Certain poses may require adjustments to accommodate the physical changes in your body and a heightened state of stress that many people experience during perimenopause. Here are some of my suggestions for modifications.

Modifications for forward folds

If you have osteoporosis, avoid deep forward folds (flexion) with a rounded spine. For example, in a standing or seated forward fold (uttanasana and paschimottanasana), bend your knees and rest your ribs on your thighs, spine straight. This is also a good modification if you have hot flushes, headaches, glaucoma or dizziness, because it keeps your head level with your heart. It prevents blood rushing towards your head, which could trigger all of those symptoms just listed.

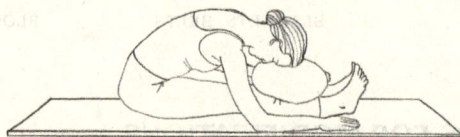

SEATED FORWARD FOLD (PASCHIMOTTANASANA), WITH BOLSTER

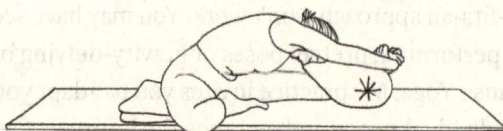

SEATED HEAD TO KNEE FORWARD FOLD (JANUSIRSASANA), WITH BOLSTER

Instead of this deep flexion in seated forward fold pose (paschimottanasana and janusirsasana), practise a modified version instead, with the forehead supported on a low bolster (pictured) or a high upturned bolster, or rest forehead and arms on a chair (pictured).

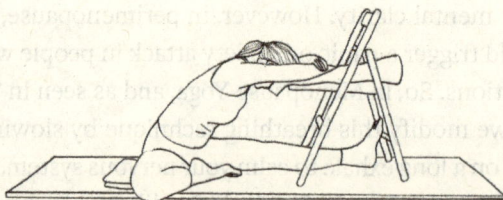

SEATED HEAD TO KNEE FORWARD FOLD (JANUSIRSASANA), WITH CHAIR

In a standing forward fold (uttanasana) or downward facing dog pose (adho mukha svanasana) use bricks, a chair, bolster or a wall to maintain a straight spine, including your neck.

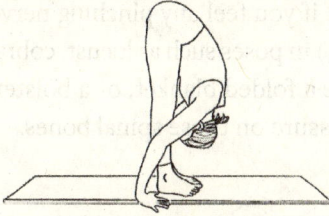

STANDING FORWARD FOLD
(UTTANASANA)

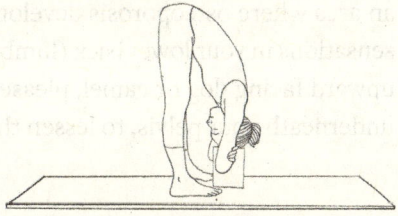

STANDING FORWARD FOLD
(UTTANASANA), WITH BRICK

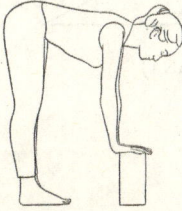

FORWARD FOLD
(MODIFIED UTTANASANA)

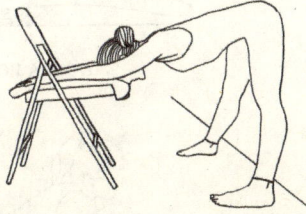

WIDE-LEGGED STANDING FORWARD
FOLD (MODIFIED PADOTTANASANA),
WITH WALL OR CHAIR SUPPORT

Modifications for balance poses

Beginners who are building balance and leg strength can swap the traditional warrior 3 pose (virabhadrasana III) for a modified version resting hands on bricks.

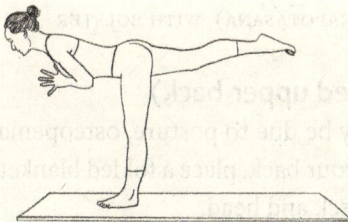

WARRIOR 3 POSE
(VIRABHADRASANA III),
WITHOUT PROPS

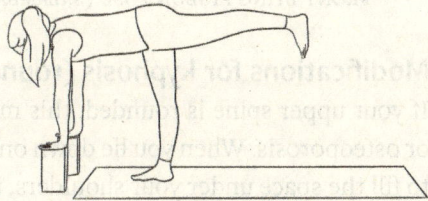

WARRIOR 3 POSE
(MODIFIED VIRABHADRASANA III),
WITH BRICKS

Modifications for lower back compression

The vertebral discs in our lower back may become compressed over time and cause deterioration in our lumbar spine bones due to sitting at desks, driving long distance, age and the menopause. Your lumbar spine may be an area where osteoporosis develops. So, if you feel any pinching nerve sensations in your lower back (lumbar 4–5) in poses such as locust, cobra, upward facing dog or camel, please place a folded blanket, or a bolster, underneath your pelvis, to lessen the pressure on those spinal bones.

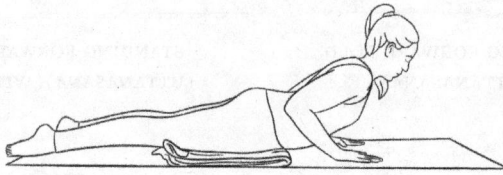

COBRA POSE (BHUJANGASANA)

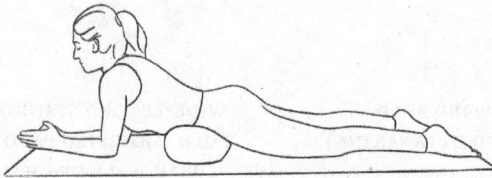

SPHINX POSE (MODIFIED SALAMBA BHUJANGASANA), WITH BOLSTER

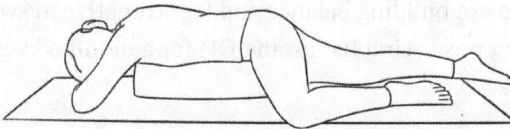

FRONT LYING PIGEON POSE (SALAMBA KAPOTASANA), WITH BOLSTER

Modifications for kyphosis (rounded upper back)

If your upper spine is rounded, this may be due to posture, osteopenia or osteoporosis. When you lie down on your back, place a folded blanket to fill the space under your shoulders, neck and head.

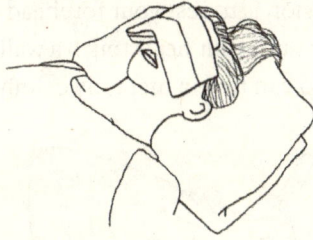

RELAXATION POSE WITH EYE CLOTH AND HEAD SUPPORT

When lying on the front of your body in spine extension poses such as cobra and locust, avoid arching your neck. Keep your neck straight, look to the floor and use your upper back muscles to lift your chest.

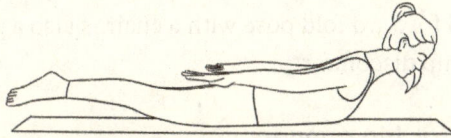

LOCUST POSE (SALABASANA), ARMS BACK, NECK LONG

If your upper back rounds and shoulders feel tight in downward facing dog pose (adho mukha svanasana), place your hands on bricks to create more space for your spine to lengthen. This also helps if you have a long legs to shorter torso ratio. Alternatively, place your hands at the wall.

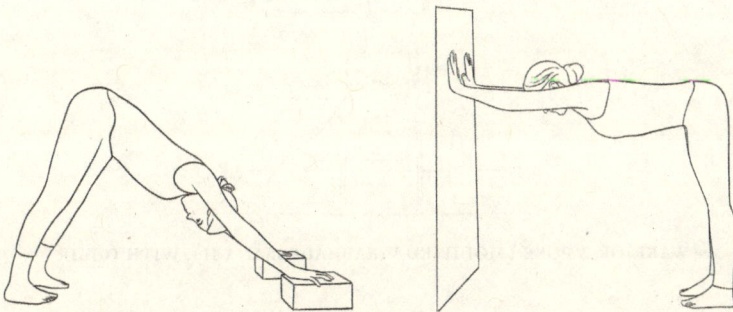

DOWNWARD FACING DOG POSE (ADHO MUKHA SVANASANA)

Downward facing dog pose (adho mukha svanasana) is good for a spine and hamstring leg stretch, but without pressure on the shoulders or wrists. The variation with bricks is also suitable for people with hot flushes, migraine headaches, dizziness, high or low blood pressure or glaucoma. Another version is to rest your forehead on the edge of a chair and walk your feet back until your heels touch a wall. This is a more stable version of this pose and can have a mentally calming effect.

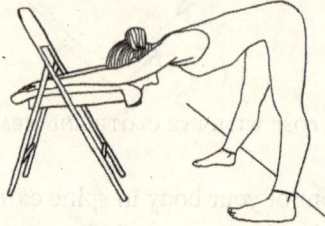

STANDING WIDE-LEGGED FORWARD FOLD
(PRASARITA PADOTTANASANA), WITH CHAIR

This wide-legged forward fold pose with a chair is also a good modification if you have hip discomfort.

Modifications for hip openers

If you are experiencing discomfort in your hip sockets due to inflammation, consider sitting on a chair in poses such as warrior 2 (virabhadrasana II), hold on to a chair during wide-legged forward fold (prasarita padottanasana), and take a narrower stance with your legs.

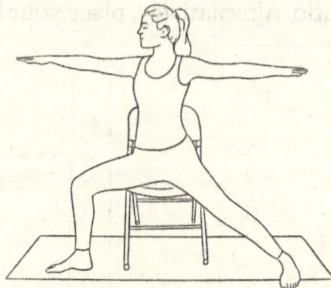

WARRIOR 2 POSE (MODIFIED VIRABHADRASANA II), WITH CHAIR

You can also use the chair to support your hips in warrior 2 pose (virabhadrasana II), triangle pose (trikonasana) and extended side angle pose (utthita parshvakonasana).

Modifications for inversions (shoulder stands, leg raised)

If you have osteopenia or osteoporosis, a shoulder stand (sarvangasana) may put dangerous strain on your neck and cervical vertebrae. I recommend you practise with legs raised on a chair with head and neck support. This is gentler and places no strain on your neck.

Even if you don't have osteoporosis, I recommend that you practise a supported shoulder stand using a brick for support, with your neck straight to avoid extra weight on your cervical spine.

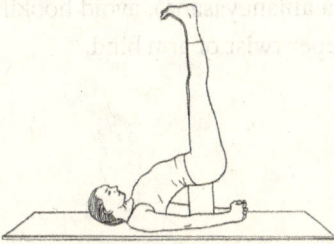

SUPPORTED SHOULDER STAND
(MODIFIED SARVANGASANA),
WITH BRICK

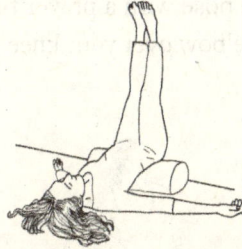

LEGS UP THE WALL POSE
(VIPARITA KARANI), WITH BOLSTER

If inversions cause your legs to go numb or give you 'pins and needles', avoid practising legs raised straight against a wall as a restorative pose, and avoid raising your pelvis up too high on a high bolster, which may also cause blood throbbing in your neck and head.

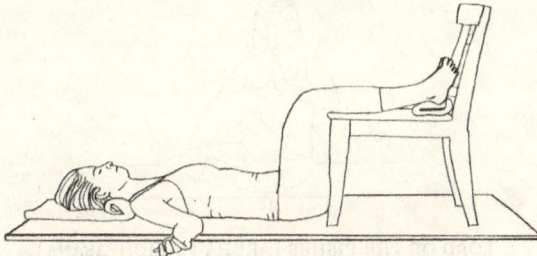

LEGS RAISED ON A CHAIR (SALAMBA SAVASANA)

Instead, replace the bolster with a folded blanket, and instead of straightening your legs against the wall, try bending your legs so your feet are touching the wall or, better still, rest your legs instead onto a chair, sofa or coffee table covered with a blanket for comfort. These modified versions allow you to *comfortably* stay longer in the restorative pose, which is more restful and refreshing.

Modifications for twists with arm binds

If you have osteoporosis, a slipped or herniated disc or lumbar spine strain, avoid unsupported twists. For example, when in a lying twist, place a brick between your legs. In a chair pose (utkatasana), seated twist or a lunge pose with a prayer twist (parivrtta anjaneyasana), avoid hooking your elbow over your knee to force a deeper twist of arm bind.

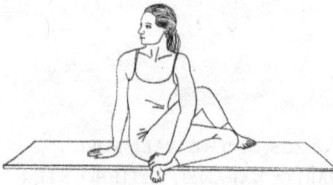

LORD OF THE FISHES OR SAGE
POSE (ARDHA MARICHYASANA/
MATSEYANDRASANA)

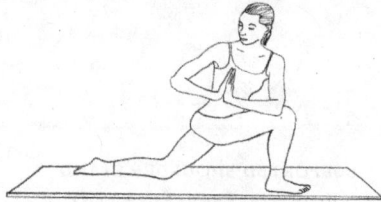

LOW LUNGE TWIST
(PARIVRTTA ANJANEYASANA),
PRAYER TWIST

Instead, use your abdominal muscles to rotate your spine naturally; you'll become stronger and increase your mobility over time.

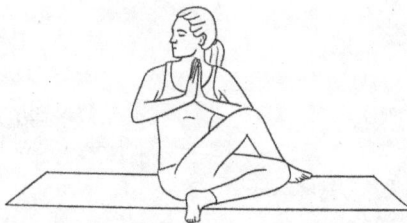

LORD OF THE FISHES (ARDHA MARICHYASANA),
PRAYER TWIST, WITHOUT USING ARMS

In chair pose (utkatasana), instead of a prayer twist, practise an open arm spine rotation that engages your abdominal muscles more.

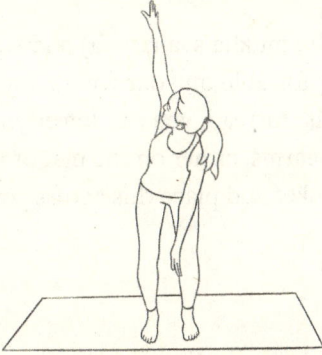

CHAIR POSE TWIST (MODIFIED
UTKATASANA), WITH OPEN ARMS

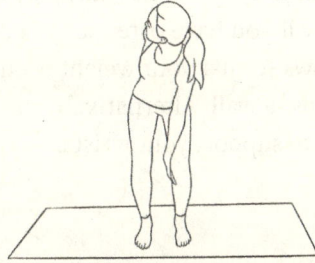

CHAIR POSE OPEN TWIST
(MODIFIED UTKATASANA), WITH
FROZEN SHOULDER ARM POSITION

If you have lower back pain in a lying twist pose, try a windshield wiper twist (supta parivrtta sucirandhrasana) with your knees progressively lowering gently from left to right side. You can also rest your legs on a cushion or bolster on one side for a supported lying twist that enables you to stay in the pose for longer, which is beneficial for digestion and easing menstrual cramps.

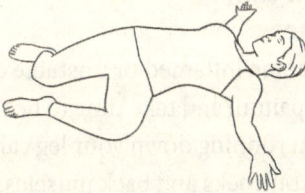

WINDSHIELD WIPER TWIST POSE
(SUPTA PARIVRTTA SUCIRANDHRASANA)

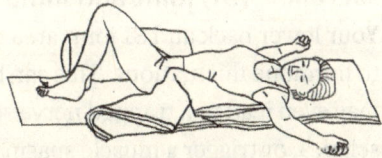

RESTORATIVE SUPPORTED
LYING TWIST POSE
(SALAMBA SUPTA MATSEYANDRASANA)

Modifications for frozen shoulder

If you have inflamed tissues in your shoulder preventing a full range of movement, avoid raising your arm above your shoulder until the inflammation eases. Instead, you can simply rest that arm alongside your body in poses with arms raised, such as sun salutations (surya namaskar), warrior 2 (virabhadrasana II), triangle (trikonasana) or tree pose (vrksasana), or place that hand at your heart for a gesture of self-kindness.

Modifications for sore wrists

Poses such as downward facing dog (adho mukha svanasana) and side plank pose (vasisthasana) may be uncomfortable on your wrists, especially if you have osteoporosis or arthritis. Instead, you can lower your elbows so that your weight is on your forearms, either on the mat or up against a wall. Alternatively, roll up a blanket and place this across your mat to support your wrists.

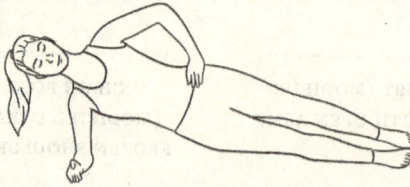

FOREARM SIDE PLANK POSE

Modifications for sore knees

In bent knee poses such as child's pose (balasana), you can lie on your back hugging a bolster instead, or with your feet against a wall with an eye bag pillow.

Modifications for pelvis instability in the sacroiliac (SI) joint and lumbar spine

Your lower back and SI joint area may become inflamed or unstable due to hormone fluctuations. This can be very painful and take time to heal. It may even lead to a trapped nerve sensation running down your leg called sciatica, or trigger a muscle spasm in your buttocks and back muscles. So please try to keep your pelvis stable, especially in longer-held yin-style poses such as pigeon pose (salamba kapotasana) and lying twists. Use a block or a bolster to level out your pelvis in pigeon pose and maintain a straight spine and neck. You may also like to rest your arms and forehead on a bolster or chair.

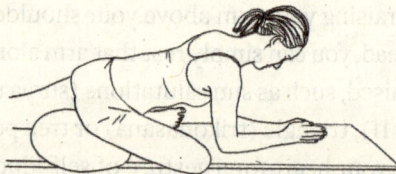

SUPPORTED PIGEON POSE (SALAMBA KAPOTASANA), WITH BOLSTER

Modifications for breathwork

If you have anxiety and panic attacks since perimenopause, slow down the breathing exercises to half the speed. This is because fast-paced repetitive breathing could trigger panic attacks. Avoid breath retention (kumbhaka) – long-held pauses in your breath. And always give yourself permission to stop the breathing technique whenever you want or need to. You can come back to the practice another day.

Modifications for trauma and hypersensitivity

In my instructions, I often suggest closing your eyes. However, if this does not feel safe or right for you, then open your eyes but aim your gaze low to the floor to avoid the light stimulating your eyes.

Modifications for vulnerability

Some of the poses include restorative postures where the hips, chest and pelvic area are held in an open stretch. If this feels too vulnerable for you to stay in these poses, you can either place a folded, heavy blanket over these parts of your body, or simply stop practising the pose.

These are just a few of the modifications for Menopause Yoga, but the best thing to do is listen to your own body. Trust yourself. If it feels good, then you are doing it right. Watch this video to see some suggested modifications you can make to your yoga poses if you have osteoporosis.[*]

Please note: you are recommended to seek advice from a health professional before undertaking movement and exercise if you have an osteoporosis diagnosis.

---

[*] https://www.youtube.com/playlist?list=PLJ-mltZchfBB9d6nOWWnOCaYHP4aQDOWC

Yoga basics:
Main poses (asanas)

STANDING POSES

MOUNTAIN POSE (MODIFIED URDHVA TADASANA)

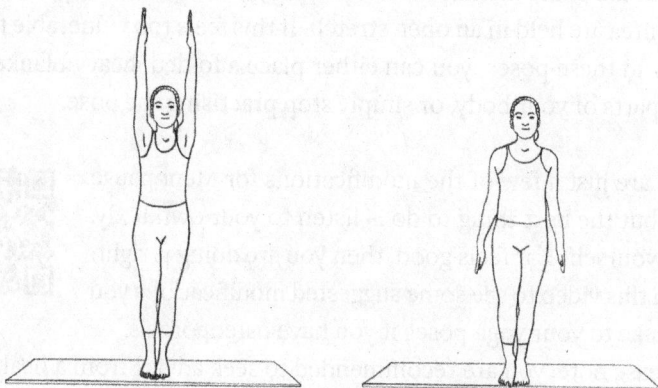

MOUNTAIN POSE (MODIFIED URDHVA TADASANA)

Stand with your feet together (or hip distance apart if more comfortable) and straighten your legs, lengthen your spine, root down into the soles of your feet, lift the crown of your head up. Relax your shoulders down your back, relax your face muscles and lower jaw. Imagine you are a mountain, strong and stable in your stature.

TREE POSE (VRKSASANA)

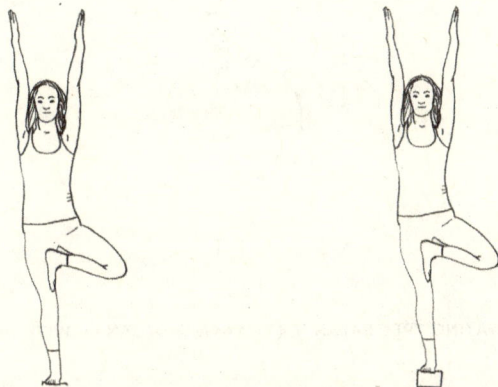

TREE POSE (VRKSASANA)

1. Stand on your right leg, raise your left knee, use your hand to open your hip and place the sole of your left foot on the inside of your right thigh or inside shin or ankle. Never place the foot on your knee as it could destabilize your knee joint.
2. Focus your eye gaze on something directly in front of you. Breathe slowly for 10 breaths before slowly lowering the left foot to the floor.
3. Set a timer for 10 breaths, approximately 1 minute on each leg.

Challenge: Stand on a wood or cork yoga brick. Make sure your heel is on the brick, but your toes can be off the brick. Do not stand on foam blocks as they are not stable. See if you can sway your body side to side and still regain balance.

Tip: To build confidence, place one hand on a wall or chair. Next, place the palms of both hands together and press together with equal force. This helps to balance the left and right side of your body.

Modification: Standing on a wood or cork yoga brick, place your hand on a chair or a wall for balance while you get used to this added balance. You may wobble at the start, but this is just your feet muscles responding to the new challenge, which is good.

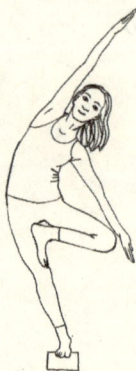

SWAYING TREE BALANCE (TIRYAKA TADASANA), WITH BRICK

STANDING PIGEON POSE (TADA KAPOTASANA)

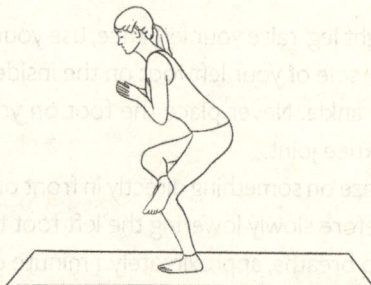

STANDING PIGEON POSE (TADA KAPOTASANA)

1. Start in tree pose (vrksasana), standing on your left leg. Then slide your right foot across your left thigh (above the knee) and bend your standing leg, as if sitting down in a chair.
2. Place the palms of the hands together in a prayer mudra. Lengthen your tailbone back and the crown of your head forward, so that your spine feels straight.
3. Stay for 5–10 breaths balancing on your left leg, and then stand up and change to balance on your right leg for 5–10 breaths.

Beginners: Hold on to a chair or wall in front of you for balance.

Challenge: Sit deeper into the imaginary chair and reach your arms forward for a balance challenge, or lower your hands down to the mat for a deeper glute muscle stretch.

CHAIR POSE (UTKATASANA)

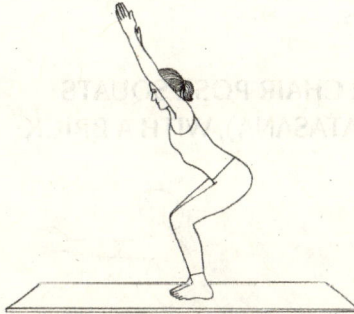

CHAIR POSE (UTKATASANA)

1. Stand with your legs together, and then sit down into an imaginary chair. Put the weight into your heels and check you can see your toes in front of your knees. (There is an option to raise your arms forward or above your head.)

2. Stay for 5 breaths. Then stand up into mountain pose (tadasana).

CHAIR POSE (MODIFIED UTKATASANA), WITH BRICK AND HEEL LIFTS

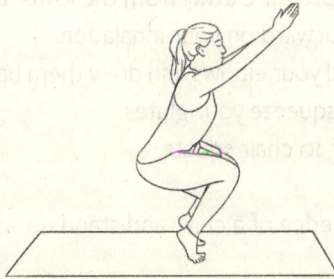

CHAIR POSE (MODIFIED UTKATASANA), WITH A BRICK AND HEEL LIFTS

1. From standing, place a brick between your thighs and lift the heels of both feet off the floor.

2. Bend your knees as if sitting into a chair and reach your arms forward to help you balance.

3. Inhale as you slowly straighten your legs (keep your heels lifted), and ·

exhale as you lower your heels. Squeezing the brick will help you balance and engage your pelvic floor and abdominal muscles too.

4. Repeat 5–10 times.

MENO-WARRIOR CHAIR POSE SQUATS (MODIFIED UTKATASANA), WITH A BRICK

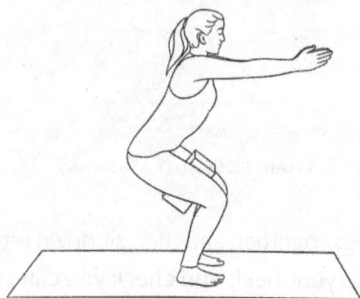

CHAIR POSE (MODIFIED UTKATASANA), WITH A BRICK AND ARMS FORWARD

1. Stand with your feet hip distance apart and place a brick between your mid-thighs.
2. Bend your knees as if sitting back into a chair. Squeeze the block to engage your leg muscles. This also prevents your knees from dropping inwards and takes pressure away from the lower back.
3. Reach your arms forward on your inhalation.
4. As you exhale, bend your elbows and draw them back towards your ribs, stand upright and squeeze your glutes.
5. Repeat 3 rounds of 10 chair squats.

Beginners: Sit on the edge of a chair and stand up 10 times without using your arms to lift you.

CHAIR POSE SQUATS (MODIFIED UTKATASANA), WITH A BRICK AND PULSING

1. Squeeze the brick between your thighs as you make tiny pulsing movements up and down (2–4cm (approx. 1–1.5 inches) only).
2. Practise three rounds of 10 pulses and then stand in mountain pose (tadasana) for a few breaths.
3. Repeat 2–3 rounds of 10 pulses.

4. Hold the chair pose squat for 10 slow breaths, and then stand in mountain pose (tadasana).

Tip: Placing weight into your heels takes pressure off your knees.

Challenge: Hold a heavy-weight dumbbell in your hands, close to your chest, as you pulse. Start with 1–2kgs (approx. 3–4lbs) and increase the weight over time.

WARRIOR 3 POSE (MODIFIED VIRABHADRASANA III)

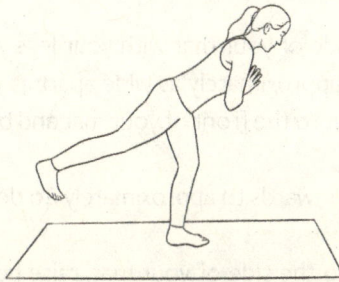

WARRIOR 3 POSE (MODIFIED VIRABHADRASANA III)

1. Start in chair pose squat (modified utkatasana). Place your hands on your hips to make sure they stay level with the floor.
2. Straighten your left leg behind you and keep your right leg bent.
3. Lift your back foot off the floor – just 2–4cm (approx. 1–1.5 inches). Pulse up and down with your standing leg 5–10 times, to strengthen your glute and thigh muscles.
4. Sit into chair pose (utkatasana) with both legs.
5. Stand up into mountain pose (tadasana) for a few breaths before returning to chair pose (utkatasana) and balancing on your left leg, pulsing 5–10 times. Then stand in mountain pose (tadasana).

Beginners: Wobbling is good – it means you are activating your leg, foot and ankle muscles to build balance. Start by resting your hands at a wall or on a chair to build confidence.

WARRIOR 2 POSE (VIRABHADRASANA II)

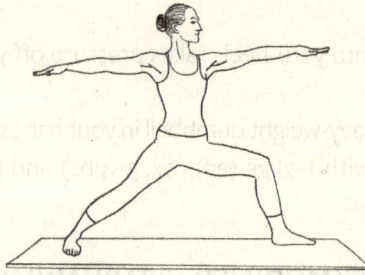

WARRIOR 2 POSE (VIRABHADRASANA II)

1. Stand facing the side of your mat with your legs wide apart and check that your feet are approximately as wide apart as your hands.
2. Turn your right foot to the front of your mat and bend your knee above your ankle.
3. Turn your left foot inwards to approximately 40 degrees (avoid twisting your kneecap).
4. Open your chest to the side of your mat, raise both arms to shoulder height and look at the middle finger of your right hand.
5. Stay for 10 slow breaths.
6. Then turn to face the other side of your mat in warrior 2 pose (virabhadrasana II), with your left foot turned forward.

Modifications for frozen or sore shoulder: Place the hand of the affected arm on your chest so you can feel your heartbeat. If you have a tight neck and upper back muscles, turn the palms of your hands upwards and allow your shoulder blades to relax.

Modifications for hip discomfort: Practise with narrow leg stance or sit on a chair (see 'Modifications for hip openers').

GODDESS HIGH SQUAT POSE (UTKATA KONASANA)

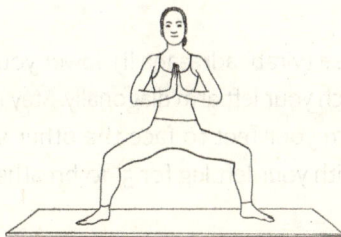

GODDESS HIGH SQUAT POSE (UTKATA KONASANA)

1. Stand with the feet wide, toes turned out, heels turned in.
2. Bend your knees so your kneecaps track above your 2nd toe. Check your arches are lifted and not collapsing. Your hands are in prayer or Goddess Hakini mudra.
3. Inhale, straighten your legs and raise your arms.
4. Exhale, bend your knees into a squat again and bend your elbows.

Option: Add lion's breath (simhasana pranayama) to release anger or emotional tension.

EXTENDED TRIANGLE POSE (UTTHITA TRIKONASANA)

1. Step your feet wide apart and turn your right foot to the front of your mat. Turn the back foot to 40 degrees.
2. Open your arms wide and lengthen from your waist sideways, and then lower your right hand down to your shin bone or a block.
3. Raise your left arm up and draw your lower ribs in. Stay for 5–10 breaths.
4. Come upright and turn your feet to the other side of the mat with your left foot in front. Repeat the pose.

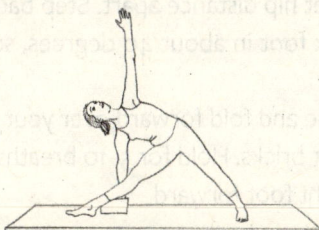

EXTENDED TRIANGLE POSE (UTTHITA TRIKONASANA)

EXTENDED SIDE ANGLE POSE (UTTHITA PARSVAKONASANA)

1. From warrior 2 pose (virabhadrasana II), lower your right elbow to your right thigh and reach your left arm diagonally. Stay here for 5–10 breaths.
2. Come upright, turn your feet to face the other side of your mat and repeat the pose with your left leg for 5–10 breaths.

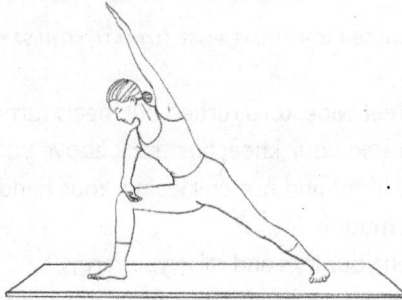

EXTENDED SIDE ANGLE POSE (UTTHITA PARSVAKONASANA)

Challenge: Lower your right hand inside your right foot, or on a block, or bind your right arm underneath your right leg.

PYRAMID POSE (PARSVOTTANASANA)

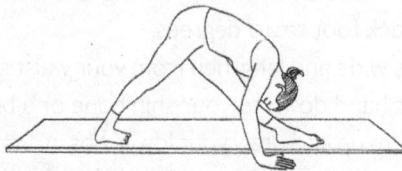

PYRAMID POSE (PARSVOTTANASANA)

1. Stand with your feet hip distance apart. Step back with your right foot and turn your back foot in about 40 degrees, so your hips are facing forward.
2. Lengthen your spine and fold forward over your left leg, lowering your hands to the mat or bricks. Hold for 5–10 breaths.
3. Repeat with the right foot forward.

Modifications for osteopenia and tight hamstrings: Place your hands on the bricks with your spine straight.

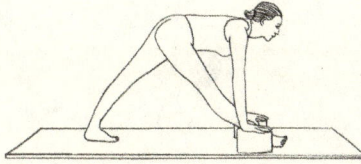

PYRAMID POSE (PARSVOTTANASANA) MODIFIED, WITH BRICKS

Modifications for hot flushes and headaches: Keep your head level with your heart.

LOW CRESCENT LUNGE (ANJANEYASANA)

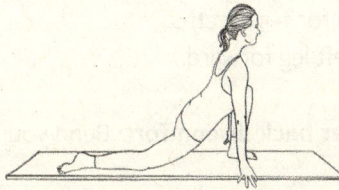

LOW CRESCENT LUNGE (ANJANEYASANA)

1. Kneel on your mat with your hands under your shoulders and knees under your hips in table top pose (bharmanasana).
2. From table top pose (bharmanasana) (hands and knees position), step your right foot forward.
3. Stay for 1–5 breaths, then return to table top pose (bharmanasana).
4. Step your left foot forward and raise your arms.

HIGH CRESCENT LUNGE (ASHTA CHANDRASANA)

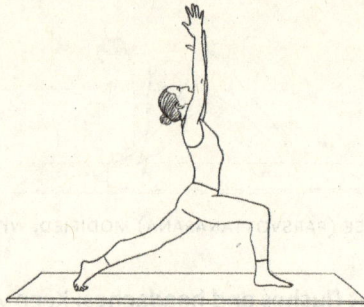

HIGH CRESCENT LUNGE (ASHTA CHANDRASANA)

1. Stand with feet hip distance apart, step back with your left foot, keep the back heel lifted and bend your right knee.
2. Raise your arms up for 1–5 breaths.
3. Repeat with your left leg forward.

Modification for lower back discomfort: Bend your back knee and tuck your tailbone slightly.

SIDE LUNGE (SKANDASANA)

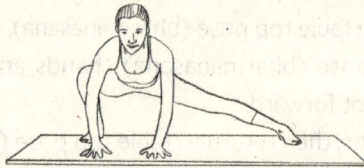

SIDE LUNGE (SKANDASANA)

1. From high crescent lunge (ashta chandrasana) or low crescent lunge (anjaneyasana), turn to the side of your mat with one knee bent and the other leg straight.
2. Shift your weight from your right to your left side, to stretch your inner thighs.

Modifications for hip discomfort: Narrow your leg width and place your hands on a chair, bolster or bricks for support as you shift gently side to side.

Modifications for knee pain: Avoid side lunges (skandasana) and practise standing wide-legged forward fold (prasarita padottanasana) instead.

BACKBENDS AND SPINE MOBILITY POSES

CAT-COW (MARJARYASANA-BITILASANA) FLOW

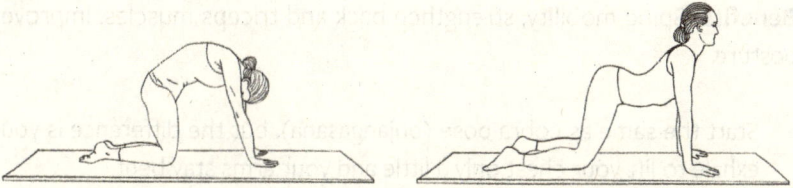

CAT POSE (MARJARYASANA) AND COW POSE (BITILASANA) FLOW

1. From all fours in table top pose (bharmanasana), press your hands and feet into the mat so your limbs support your spine. Initiate the spinal movement from your tailbone and not your head.
2. Inhale, lift your tailbone and move sequentially through your spine as you dip your back and open across your chest. Look forward and lift your chin.
3. Exhale, lower your tailbone and round your back, drawing your navel in and up, allowing your head to lower.
4. Repeat these flowing flexion (arching) and extension (rounding) spine movements with your breath.
5. Close your eyes to develop interoception (inner body awareness).

COBRA POSE (BUJANGASANA) WITH BLANKET

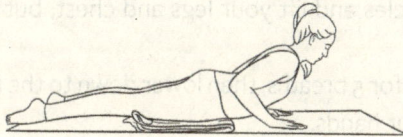

COBRA POSE (BUJANGASANA)

Benefits: A chest stretch that invites deeper breathing and improves spine posture.

1. Start lying on the front of your body with your hands at the sides of your ribs, elbows bent.
2. Inhale as you lift your chest forward and up, straightening your arms a little.
3. Exhale as you lower your chest.

LOW COBRA POSE LIFTS (MODIFIED BUJANGASANA)

Benefits: Spine mobility, strengthen back and triceps muscles, improve posture.

1. Start the same as cobra pose (bujangasana), but the difference is you exhale to lift your chest only a little and your arms stay bent.
2. Press into your hands and attempt to slide them back. Inhale as you lower onto the mat and turn your head to one side.
3. Repeat 10 times, alternating your head turn.

LOCUST POSE (SALABHASANA)

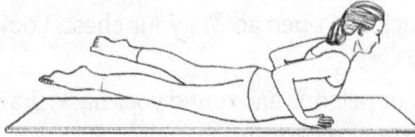

LOCUST POSE (SALABHASANA), BEGINNER'S VERSION

Benefits: Spine mobility, strengthens back and triceps muscles, improves posture.

1. Start in low cobra pose (modified bujangasana). Exhale to engage your abdominal muscles and lift your legs and chest, but keep your hands on the mat.
2. Stay in the pose for 5 breaths, then lower down to the mat and rest your forehead on your hands.

LOCUST POSE (SALABHASANA), WITH ARMS LIFTED

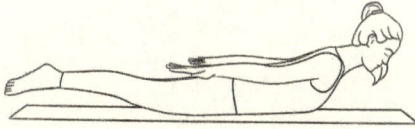

LOCUST POSE (SALABHASANA)

1. Start with the beginner's version of locust pose, then lift your arms, reaching your hands back in an arrow shape.
2. Stay for 5 breaths.

Modification for lower back: Place a folded blanket under your abdomen (see 'Modifications for lower back compression').

SUPPORTED CAMEL POSE (USTRASANA)

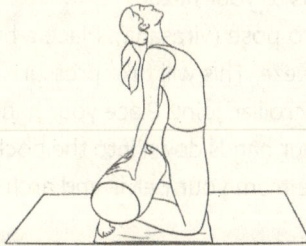

SUPPORTED CAMEL POSE (MODIFIED USTRASANA)

1. From kneeling position, squeeze a brick between your thighs and place a bolster behind your heels.
2. Centre your pelvis over your knees and slide your hands down your pelvis until they touch the bolster behind you.
3. Look up, but avoid throwing your head back. Exhale, engage your core muscles to reverse out of the pose, lower your chin to your chest and sit back into a kneeling hero pose (virasana).

CAMEL POSE (USTRASANA), FULL OPTION

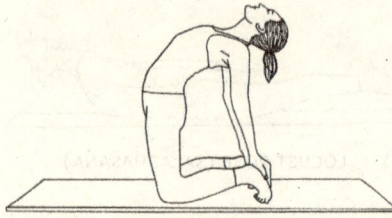

CAMEL POSE (USTRASANA)

Benefits: Chest stretches (heart lifts) invite deeper breath, may lift low mood and re-energize, and may relieve headaches. Spine extension may strengthen spine muscles for posture. This may benefit people with hyper-kyphosis and osteopenia.

1. Start in supported camel pose (ustrasana), then roll the bolster away and lower your hands to your heels.
2. Start in kneeling hero pose (virasana). Place a brick or block between your thighs and squeeze. This will take pressure off your lumbar spine and stabilize your sacroiliac joint. Place your hands at the back of your pelvis, as if sliding your hands down into the pockets of tight jeans.
3. Lengthen your spine from your pelvis and arch your spine to stretch your chest.
4. Look forward or up to the ceiling, but avoid throwing your head back, as this can compress your neck (contraindicated for osteoporosis).

Beginners: Sit at the front of a bolster and reach your hands to the back of the bolster for support. This will alleviate pressure on the lumbar spine.

BRIDGE POSE (SETU BANDHA SARVANGASANA)

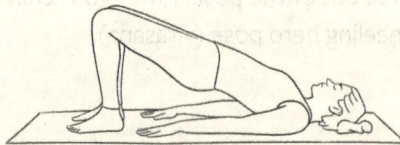

BRIDGE POSE (SETU BANDHA SARVANGASANA)

Benefits: Heart opening pose that lifts energy, shifts lethargy, deepens breathing and invites a positive mindset.

1. Start lying on your back with your knees bent and feet on the mat, feet and knees hip distance apart. Combine pelvic floor tilts with small incremental movements lifting through your spine 1cm (approx. 0.5 inch), or one vertebra at a time. Always move your spine on the exhalation to engage your core muscles.
2. Repeat these movements 6–8 times, until you are on your shoulder blades, but keep your spine straight so you can still see your knees.

BRIDGE POSE (MODIFIED SETU BANDHA SARVANGASANA), WITH LEG LIFT

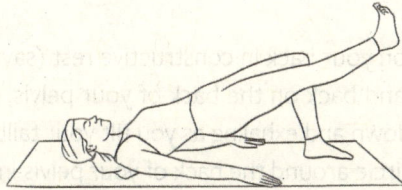

BRIDGE POSE (MODIFIED SETU BANDHA SARVANGASANA)

Benefits: Strengthens glute and legs muscles.

1. Start in bridge pose (setu bandha sarvangasana), but straighten one leg forward at the same height as your knees.
2. Option to either stay in static hold for 5–10 breaths or pulse up and down 10 times.

HALF AND FULL BOW POSE (DANURASANA)

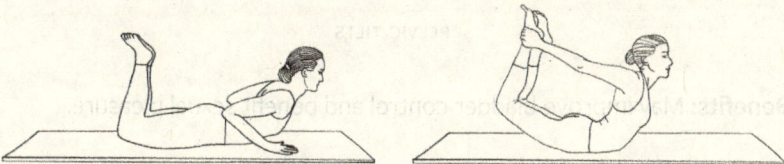

HALF AND FULL BOW POSE (DANURASANA)

Benefits: Spine flexibility, may ease bloating.

1. Start in cobra pose (bujangasana), then bend your knees and lift your feet. Check there is no back pain, then relax onto the mat.
2. Reach your hands back to hold the outside edges of your feet, but keep your head on the mat. As you exhale, engage your abdominal muscles and push your feet away. This will lift your chest and head off the mat.
3. Stay for a few breaths and then release and relax onto the mat.

PELVIC FLOOR POSES

PELVIC CIRCLES

These can be done clockwise and anticlockwise, on your hands and knees, or lying on your back.

1. Begin by lying on your back in constructive rest (savasana).
2. Rock forward and back on the back of your pelvis, inhaling as you tilt your tailbone down and exhaling as you tilt your tailbone up.
3. Then start to circle around the back of your pelvis in a clockwise direction, without lifting your pelvis off the mat. Repeat 8–10 times. You may notice the muscles in your lower abdomen start to work! Then rotate in an anticlockwise direction, 8–10 times.
4. Relax. Pelvic tone comes from the ability to engage and relax these muscles.

PELVIC TILTS, WITH BRICK OR BLOCK

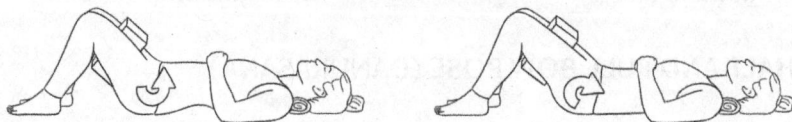

PELVIC TILTS

Benefits: May improve bladder control and benefit sexual pleasure.

1. Start lying on your back in constructive rest (savasana).
2. Place a brick or block between your thighs and squeeze to engage your pelvic floor, leg and glute muscles.

3. Rock forward and back on the back of your pelvis, inhaling as you tilt your tailbone down and exhaling as you tilt your tailbone up.

4. Visualize a rose flower at the base of your perineum (in between your anus and vagina).

5. Inhale, tilt your tailbone down so that your lower back arches slightly, and visualize the rose petals opening as you relax your perineum.

6. Exhale, tilt your tailbone up so your lower back flattens towards the mat, and visualize the rose closing into a tight bud as you contract your perineum, lifting in and upwards towards your navel.

7. Repeat these movements 10 times with your breath and rose visualization. Then remove the brick or block and relax. Pelvic tone comes from the ability to engage and relax these muscles.

PELVIC FLOOR BRIDGE POSE

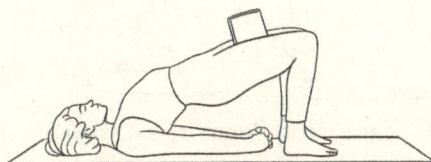

PELVIC FLOOR BRIDGE POSE (SETU BANDHA SARVANGASANA)

Benefits: Strengthens weak pelvic floor and leg muscles, chest stretch, deeper breathing. May improve bladder control and benefit sexual pleasure.

1. From constructive rest (savasana), place a yoga brick or thick block between your legs and squeeze between your mid-thighs. Make sure your feet are as wide apart as your knees.

2. Every time you exhale, incrementally roll up your spine slightly higher, inhale in a low bridge pose, and then exhale as you slowly lower down your spine, squeezing your block or brick.

3. Add the rose flower visualization from 'Pelvic tilts with brick or block'. Repeat 10 times.

4. Remove the brick or block, open your knees with the soles of your feet touching to relax your pelvic floor. Remember – healthy pelvic floor tone comes from being able to switch the muscles on and off.

Tip: To balance strength in your inner and outer glutes and thigh muscles, swap the brick for a Pilates band. Place the band half way up your thighs, come into bridge pose (setu bandha sarvangasana), inhale as you widen your knees apart and exhale to relax. Repeat 5–10 times, then lower your pelvis to the mat. Repeat the exercise 2 to 3 times. Relax and hug your knees to your chest.

Counterpose: Practise a glute stretch such as thread the needle pose (urdhva mukha pasasana) on the left and then the right leg.

FORWARD FOLDS

CHILD'S POSE (BALASANA)

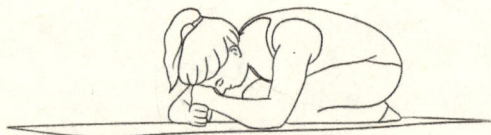

CHILD'S POSE (MODIFIED BALASANA)

Benefits: Stretches spine muscles and fascia from the neck to the tailbone. Can ease bloating and digestive gas. Resting forehead marma points (Ayurvedic acupressure points) on the hands or a brick may calm the mind, alleviating anxiety and overwhelm.

1. Kneel on the mat with your knees wide or together, depending on which is more comfortable, and fold your torso forward. Rest your forehead onto either the floor, your hands, or a block.

CHILD'S POSE WITH EXTENDED ARMS (UTTHITA BALASANA)

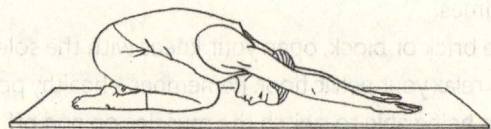

CHILD'S POSE WITH EXTENDED ARMS (UTTHITA BALASANA)

Benefits: May help alleviate lower back discomfort and menstrual cramps, stretches spine and shoulders.

1. From table top pose (bharmanasana), touch your big toes together, keep your hands where they are and straighten your arms as you sit your tailbone back towards your heels. The aim is to stretch your back muscles and relax your abdomen, so keep your arms straight.
2. Stay for 5–10 breaths.

WIDE KNEE CHILD'S POSE (UTTHITA BALASANA)

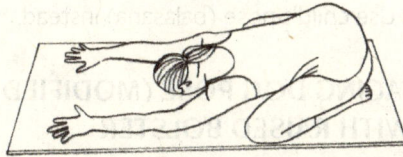

WIDE KNEE CHILD'S POSE (UTTHITA BALASANA)

Tip: To cool hot flushes, rest your forehead onto a brick or block.

Modification for knee pain: Place a folded blanket behind your kneecaps, or sit back on a bolster so your hips are higher.

DOWNWARD FACING DOG POSE (ADHO MUKHA SVANASANA)

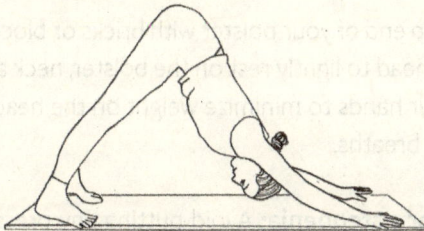

DOWNWARD FACING DOG POSE (ADHO MUKHA SVANASANA)

1. Begin in table top pose (bharmanasana) with your hands under your shoulders.
2. Lift your hips up and back, straightening your legs as much as is comfortably possible.

3. Lengthen your spine by pushing your hips back and your chest forward. Position your ears between your upper arms.

Modification for tight shoulders, hyperkyphosis, long legs with a short torso and osteopenia: Place your hands on bricks to create more space for your spine, bend your knees and place feet wider apart.

Modification for menorage: Press your heels against a wall. This can help you stay longer in the pose (see 'Modifications for kyphosis (rounded upper back)').

Alternative pose: Use child's pose (balasana) instead.

DOWNWARD FACING DOG POSE (MODIFIED ADHO MUKHA SVANASANA), WITH RAISED BOLSTER

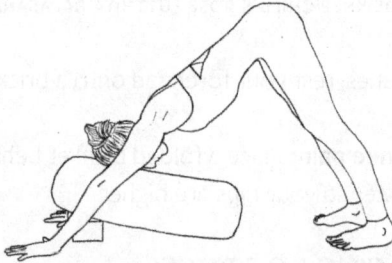

DOWNWARD FACING DOG POSE (MODIFIED ADHO MUKHA SVANASANA), WITH FOREHEAD ON RAISED BOLSTER, NECK STRAIGHT

1. Elevate the top end of your bolster with bricks or blocks to a height that enables your head to lightly rest on the bolster, neck and spine straight.
2. Press into your hands to minimize weight on the head.
3. Hold for 5-10 breaths.

Modifications for osteopenia: Avoid putting any pressure on the neck. Option to rest in supported child's pose (salamba balasana) with the bolster instead.

STANDING WIDE-LEGGED FORWARD FOLD (SALAMBA PRASARITA PADOTTANASANA)

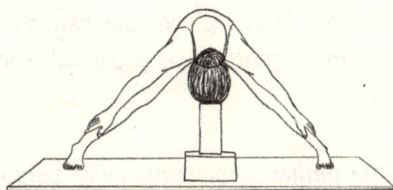

STANDING WIDE-LEGGED FORWARD FOLD (SALAMBA PRASARITA PADOTTANASANA), WITH BRICKS

Benefits: Soothes menorage and irritability, hip-opening stretch.

1. Place one or more bricks or blocks half way down your mat.
2. Step your feet wide and parallel with the sides of your mat.
3. Bend your knees and hinge forward at your hips with a straight spine.
4. Lower your head to the bricks to calm your mind. Start to straighten your legs as much as is comfortable.
5. Stay for 5–10 breaths.

Modifications: Replace bricks for softer bolsters, or practise with a chair (see 'Using props for modifications').

STANDING FORWARD FOLD (UTTANASANA)

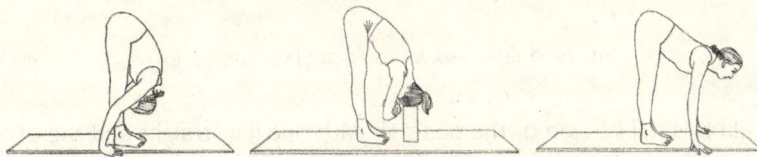

STANDING FORWARD FOLD (UTTANASANA)

1. Start in a crouching position looking forward with your hands either beside your feet, on blocks or on a chair.
2. As you exhale, start to straighten your legs but keep them bent. Rest your rib cage on your thighs.
3. As you inhale, return to a crouching position.
4. As you exhale, start to straighten your legs more, but keep your ribs resting on your thighs.

5. Repeat 5 times.
6. Stay in forward fold, either arms rag doll relaxed or hold your opposite arm and rest your elbows on bent knees. Stay for 5–10 breaths.
7. To stand up, bend your knees, place your hands on the front of your ankles and slide them up your legs as you slowly roll up your spine to a standing position.

Modification for osteopenia: Come upright with bent knees and a straight spine.

Modification for hot flushes, headaches, high or low blood pressure and glaucoma: Have your elbows and ribs resting on your thighs and your spine straight with your head level with your heart (like a table top). Stand up with a straight spine, hinging at your hips, or place your hands on a chair to stand up. (See 'Using props for modifications'.)

Tip: Keeping your hands on your legs helps in avoiding feeling dizzy.

HEAD TO KNEE FORWARD FOLD (JANUSIRSASANA)

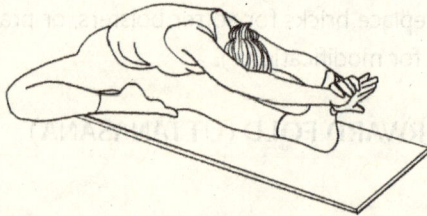

HEAD TO KNEE FORWARD FOLD (JANUSIRSASANA)

1. In this full version of the pose, sit with one leg straight and the other knee bent, with the sole of the foot pressing into your thigh.
2. Lift and lengthen your spine and reach your arms towards the straight leg as you fold forward.
3. Hold the wrist of the opposite hand or use a yoga belt across the ball of the foot.
4. Inhale, lengthen your spine, exhale, and fold over the straight leg.
5. Stay for 8–10 breaths.

Modification for tight hamstrings and lower back: Sit up on a block or folded blanket.

Modification for knee pain: Support the knee with a block or blanket.

Modification for osteoporosis and osteopenia: Keep your spine straight and lifted, and use your arms to support your torso. Practise alternative modifications using a bolster and a chair. (See 'Using props for modifications'.)

SEATED FORWARD FOLD (PASCHIMOTTANASANA)

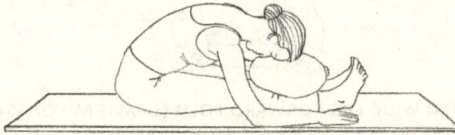

SEATED FORWARD FOLD (PASCHIMOTTANASANA)

1. Sit with straight legs and place a bolster on your shin bones.
2. Lift and lengthen your spine, then lower your torso down on top of your legs.
3. Rest your forehead on either a bolster or a brick.
4. Stay for 10 breaths. The aim is to calm your mind.

Modification for osteoporosis: Rest your forehead on an upturned bolster.

SLEEPING PIGEON POSE (EKA PADA RAJAKAPOTASANA)

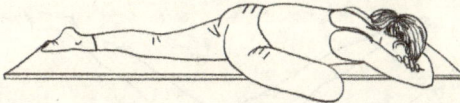

SLEEPING PIGEON POSE (EKA PADA RAJAKAPOTASANA)

Benefits: Hip and thigh stretch, relaxes glute muscles so may help with sciatica.

1. Start in table top pose (bharmanasana), then slide your right knee forward towards your wrist and the right side of the mat. Straighten your back leg.

173

2. Fold your torso forward towards the mat and rest your forehead on your hands.
3. Stay for 5–10 breaths and then return to table top pose and slide your left knee forward.

(See 'Restorative yoga poses' and 'Using props for modifications'.)

SEATED WIDE LEG FORWARD FOLD (UPAVISTA KONASANA)

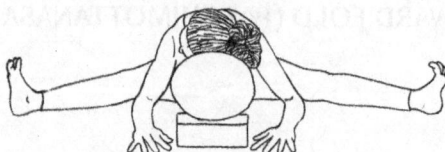

SEATED WIDE LEG FORWARD FOLD (UPAVISTA KONASANA)

1. Sit with the legs as wide as is comfortable, with your feet flexed.
2. Place your hands in front of your body and slowly lower your torso forward.

Modifications for lower back issues or tight hamstrings: Sit on a block to help tilt your pelvis forward, and place rolled-up blankets under your knees.

Modification for osteopenia: Keeping the spine straight, rest the forehead on an upturned bolster.

Alternative pose: Wide legs raised up the wall (prasarita viparita karani).

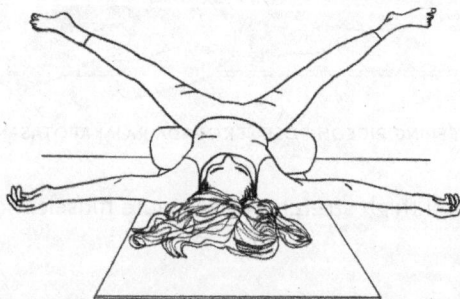

WIDE LEGS RAISED UP THE WALL (PRASARITA VIPARITA KARANI)

CORE STRENGTH POSES

TABLE TOP POSE (MODIFIED BHARMANASANA), WITH PRESS-UPS

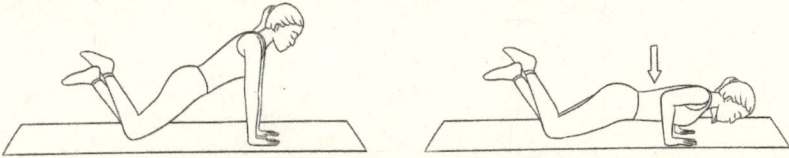

TABLE TOP POSE (MODIFIED BHARMANASANA), WITH PRESS-UPS

1. Keep your spine straight, lift your navel up towards your spine, bend your elbows and aim your chest in between your hands (not your head), 10 times, on hands and knees. Bend your elbows to 90 degree angles with your spine straight.

Modification: If you have frozen shoulder or any discomfort in your shoulders, either micro-bend your arms or avoid this exercise until your injury has healed.

BEAR POSE (BHALLUKASANA)

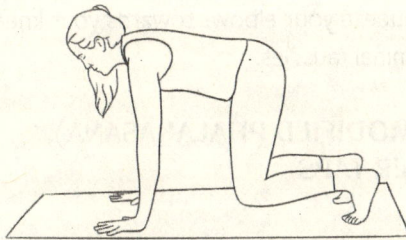

BEAR POSE (BHALLUKASANA)

This is a warm arm pose to build core strength.

1. Start in table top pose (bharmanasana) with your shoulders above your wrists and your hips above your knees.
2. Lift your knees off the floor (approx. 2 -4cm (approx. 1 -2 inches)) and hover for 5–10 breaths.

3. Every time you exhale, lift your navel towards your spine to engage your abdominal muscles.

HIGH PLANK POSE (PHALAKASANA)

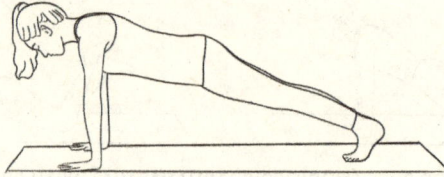

HIGH PLANK POSE (PHALAKASANA)

1. Start in bear pose (bhallukasana) and straighten both legs behind you. Every time you exhale, lift your navel towards your spine to engage your abdominal muscles. If your lower back is dipping, lift your navel more to engage your core.
2. Stay here for 10 breaths (approx. 1 minute). Set a timer and build up to 20–30 breaths (approx. 2–3 minutes).

Beginners: Start with 2 breaths and build up to 10 over time.

Modifications for wrist pain: Forearm plank or forearm plank with knees on the mat, and squeeze your elbows towards your knees to contract and engage your abdominal muscles.

PLANK POSE (MODIFIED PHALAKASANA), WITH SHOULDER TAPS

1. Start in plank pose, tap your right shoulder with your left hand, then tap your left shoulder with your right hand. Aim to not move your hips when tapping your shoulders.

Tip: Step your feet wider apart to help stabilize your pelvis.

Beginners: Stay in table top pose (bharmanasana) and tap your shoulders.

SIDE PLANK POSE (MODIFIED PHALANKASANA)

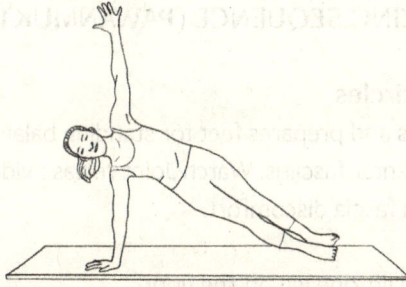

SIDE PLANK POSE (MODIFIED PHALANKASANA)

1. Start in plank pose with your feet together. Place your right hand on the centre of the mat and swivel on to the outside edge of your right foot. Option to stack your feet or step your left foot in front.
2. Raise your right arm up in line with your shoulder and chest.
3. Stay for 5–10 breaths, then change sides, with your left hand and left foot on the mat.

Beginners: Practise either the forearm-supported side plank or side plank with one leg bent.

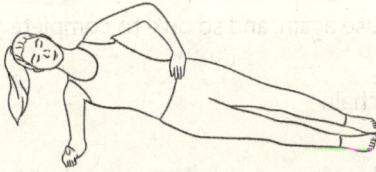

FOREARM-SUPPORTED SIDE PLANK

THREAD ARM TWISTS (VASISTHASANA HASTA PARIVRTTI)

1. Starting in a full or supported side plank pose on the right side, raise your left arm up and then slowly thread that arm underneath the lower arm. Squeeze the oblique muscles around your waist and abdomen.
2. Repeat for 10 breaths.

JOINT MOBILITY POSES

JOINT MOBILIZING SEQUENCE (PAWANMUKTASANA)

Foot and ankle circles
Benefits: Stretches and prepares feet for standing balance poses and eases plantar fasciitis. Watch Joint release video for easing joint and fascia discomfort.

1. Sit or stand and lift one leg off the floor.
2. Circle the foot clockwise a few times and then circle anticlockwise.
3. Point and flex the foot a few times.
4. Place this foot on the mat and lift all your toes.
5. Spread your toes wide. Starting with your little toe, slowly lower your toes to the mat. Notice how this foot feels more connected to the ground now.
6. Repeat on the other foot.

Foot heel raises
Benefits: Stretches and strengthens foot muscles and develops balance.

1. Raise both heels up as you inhale and lower them down as you exhale.
2. Repeat the exercise 3 times, then pause for a few seconds, do another three rounds, pause again, and so on – to complete 30 heel raises total.

Beginners: Sit on a chair.

Tip: For standing balance, raise your arms up and down.

ELBOW CIRCLES (FOR SHOULDER MOBILITY)

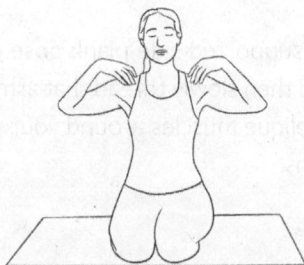

ELBOW CIRCLES

Benefits: Lubricates shoulder sockets by stimulating synovial fluid (your body's natural 'oil') with movement.

1. Place your fingertips on the front of your shoulders.
2. Inhale as you lift both elbows up and out wide. Exhale and circle your elbows back and down.
3. Add a spinal extension, arching your chest as you lift the elbows. Exhale and round your spine as you lower your elbows.
4. Repeat 5–10 times.

SHOULDER STRETCH WITH STRAP

Benefits: Stretches muscles and ligaments around the shoulders and chest.

1. Hold the strap in front of you with your hands at hip level, face down and hip distance apart.
2. Inhale, raise the strap to shoulder height, and then exhale, slowly lowering the strap.
3. Repeat the movements with the breath, incrementally lifting the strap higher until it is above your head.
4. Pause with the strap above your head, then widen your hands apart and slowly lower them behind your back.
5. Inhale as you lift the strap above your head and exhale as you lower the strap in front, to the starting position.

KNEE CIRCLES

Benefits: Mobilizes the hip joints, lubricates the hips with synovial fluid, a warm-up stretch for more wide-legged poses.

1. Lie on your back. Place your hands on your kneecaps with your legs bent, then hug knees to your chest with feet off the mat.
2. Place hands onto your kneecaps and move them in circles to lubricate your hips. Repeat 5 times clockwise and 5 times anticlockwise. Move slowly to avoid increasing heat in your body.

KNEES TO CHEST POSE (APANASANA)

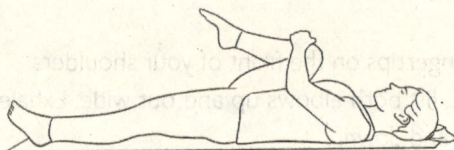

KNEES TO CHEST POSE (APANASANA)

Benefits: Hip and spine mobility, may ease lower back pain, grounding, may ease bloating and gas.

1. Inhale as you stretch your entire body, with your arms and legs extended straight.
2. Exhale slowly as you slide the sole of your right foot along the mat and bring your knee to hug your chest.
3. Repeat 10 times, alternating legs. Notice the sensation of your foot sliding along the mat, which may feel grounding. Observe your lower back gently arching with each inhale and flattening against the mat with each exhale.

HIP-OPENING POSES

Here are some other hip stretching poses with both internal and external rotation used in Menopause Yoga.

HAPPY BABY POSE (ANANDA BALASANA), FULL VERSION

There is the option to hold the ankles or the back of the knees, or hold a strap looped over the raised foot for accessibility.

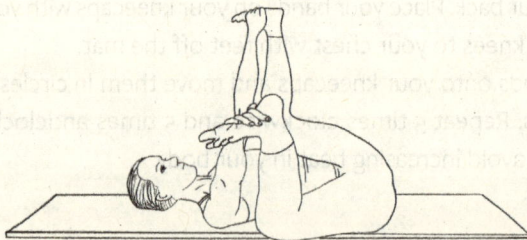

HAPPY BABY POSE (ANANDA BALASANA), FULL VERSION

LIZARD POSE (UTTHAN PRISTHASANA)

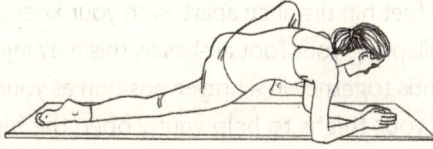

LIZARD POSE (UTTHAN PRISTHASANA)

Benefits: Hip mobility and thigh muscle stretch; may release irritability and menorage.

1. Start in a low lunge with the left foot forward.
2. Lower your arms and torso inside of your right leg.
3. Stay in the pose for 5-10 breaths.
4. Step back into table top pose (bharmanasana) with the right foot forward.

Modification for tight hips: Place your hands on bricks to bring the floor closer.

Modification for hot flushes and headaches: Keep your head level with your heart.

LOW SQUAT POSE (MALASANA)

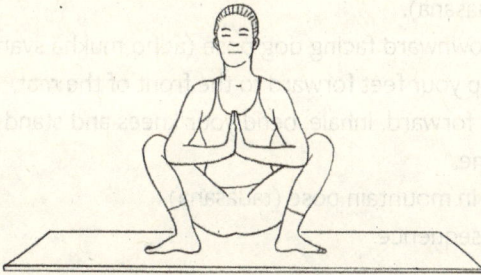

LOW SQUAT POSE (MALASANA)

Benefits: This pose may relieve constipation and gas. Do not practise it if you have diarrhoea or heavy menstruation because it can release the flow of waste or menses.

1. Start on your hands and knees in table top pose (bharmanasana).
2. Walk your hands back towards your feet into a low crouching position.
3. Separate your feet hip distance apart, with your knees in line with your toes. Avoid collapsing your foot arches as this may injure your knees.
4. Place your hands together in a prayer position at your chest with your elbows inside your thighs to help gently open the hips. Stay for 5–10 breaths.

Modification if your heels do not touch the floor: Step your feet wider apart or place a rolled towel or block under your heels.

Modification for knee joint discomfort: Sit on a raised block or bolster to support your body weight, or practise happy baby pose (ananda balasana) lying down.

SUN SALUTATION (SURYA NAMASKAR)

1. Start in mountain pose (tadasana). Inhale, and raise your arms above your head.
2. Exhale, bend your knees, hinge at your hips and fold forward. Inhale to half way, lift with a straight spine.
3. Exhale, step back to downward facing dog pose (adho mukha svanasana). Inhale to high plank pose (phalakasana).
4. Exhale, lower your body to the mat, or hover in a press-up position. Inhale to cobra pose (bujangasana) or upward facing dog pose (urdhva mukha svanasana).
5. Exhale to downward facing dog pose (adho mukha svanasana). Inhale, step or jump your feet forward to the front of the mat.
6. Exhale, fold forward. Inhale, bend your knees and stand upright with a straight spine.
7. Exhale, end in mountain pose (tadasana).
8. Repeat the sequence.

SUN SALUTATION (SURYA NAMASKAR)

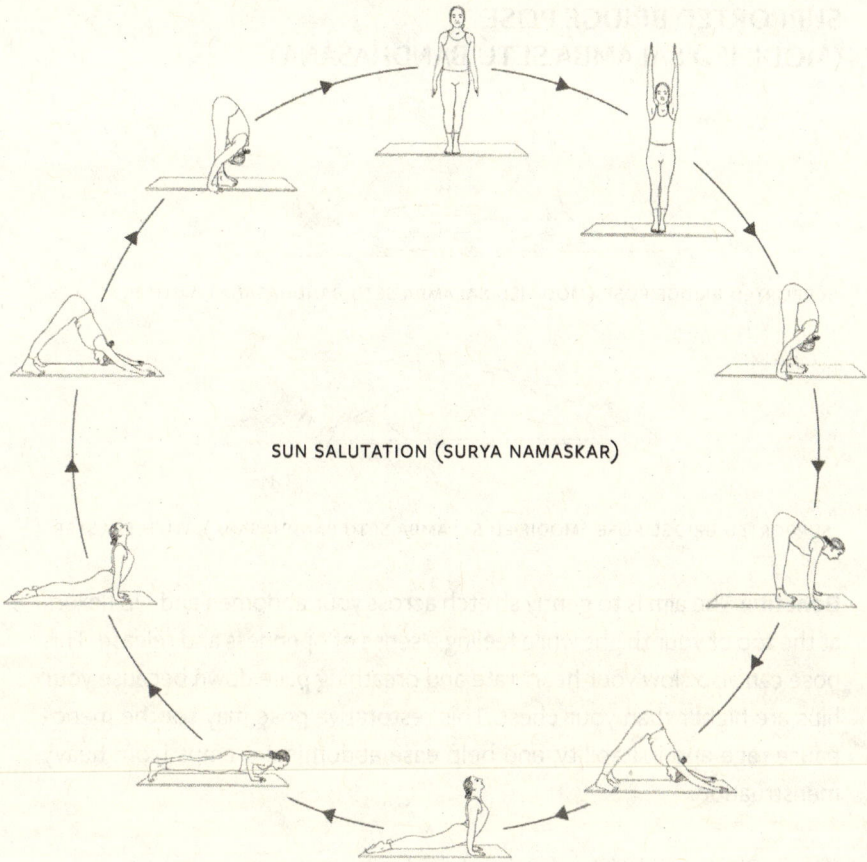

RESTORATIVE POSES

In your perimenopause I encourage you to *rest, do less, reduce stress,* to *reset* your mind, body and emotions. Menopause is your cocoon, cuddle up and enjoy nourishing and nurturing yourself. Then you'll have the energy to reemerge into your Second Spring feeling strong, healthier and happier.

Petra Coveney

SUPPORTED BRIDGE POSE
(MODIFIED SALAMBA SETU BANDHASANA)

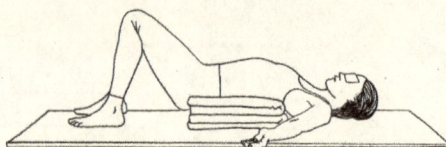

SUPPORTED BRIDGE POSE (MODIFIED SALAMBA SETU BANDHASANA), WITH BLANKETS

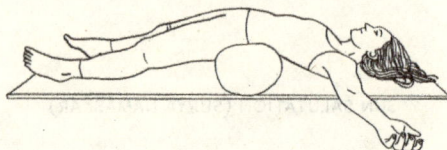

SUPPORTED BRIDGE POSE (MODIFIED SALAMBA SETU BANDHASANA), WITH BOLSTER

Benefits: The aim is to gently stretch across your abdomen and hip flexors at the top of your thighs while feeling a sense of openness and release. This pose can also slow your heart rate and breathing pace down because your hips are higher than your chest. This restorative pose may soothe menopause rage and irritability, and help ease abdominal cramps from heavy menstruation.

Props: Blanket or bolster (optional eye bag).

Coming in:

1. Place a low bolster or a folded blanket under your pelvis and lie down with your knees bent and feet on the mat. Add a blanket under your head, neck and shoulders for comfort. Open your arms to the side so your shoulder blades relax on the mat.
2. Stay for 5–10 minutes.

Modification for a deeper stretch: Straighten your legs, but avoid a pinching sensation in your lower back.

Modification for lower back discomfort: Raise your feet onto blocks or blankets or re-bend your knees with your feet flat on the mat, or lower your pelvis onto a smaller blanket.

Coming out:

1. Bend your knees and lift your hips, so you can slide the blanket or bolster forward under your knees.
2. Rest in simple relaxation pose (savasana) to neutralize your spine. The support under your knees will help relax your lower back. Stay for 5 minutes.

SUPPORTED CHILD'S POSE (SALAMBA BALASANA), WITH BOLSTER, BLOCKS AND BLANKETS

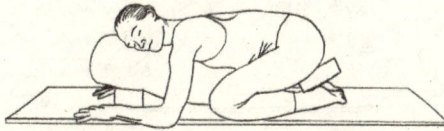

SUPPORTED CHILD'S POSE (SALAMBA BALASANA),
WITH BOLSTER, BLOCKS AND BLANKETS

Props: 1 bolster or 2 firm pillows; 1–2 bricks or blocks or a cushion; 1–2 blankets.

Coming in:

1. Set up props for a restorative child's pose (balasana). Place 1 bolster or 2 firm pillows on top of each other lengthways and 1–2 folded blanket(s) over the bolster.
2. Hug the lower end of the bolster with your knees, and then rest the front of your torso on the bolster. Adjust the bolster height to find a comfortable position.
3. If there is space between the bolster and your abdomen, fold over the blanket(s) to fill the space.
4. Rest your forearms and hands on the mat, relaxing your shoulders, or hug under the bolster.
5. Stay for 10 minutes, turning your head after 5 minutes to balance your neck stretch.

Modifications for knee discomfort: Place a folded blanket on the mat for your knees and ankles for comfort. Fold a blanket behind your knees if you feel joint discomfort.

Modification if your tailbone doesn't reach your feet: Place a block or cushion behind your heels.

Modification if the pose is uncomfortable: Come out of the pose and lie on your back with your knees bent and feet flat on the floor. You can hug a bolster or cushion for comfort.

SUPPORTED CHILD'S POSE AND 'RETREAT FROM THE WORLD' (MODIFIED SALAMBA BALASANA), WITH BLANKET

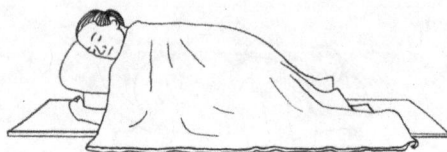

SUPPORTED CHILD'S POSE (MODIFIED SALAMBA BALASANA)
AND 'RETREAT FROM THE WORLD', WITH BLANKET

Benefits: This pose is a form of sense withdrawal (pratyahara) for times when you feel a sensory overload, overwhelm or anxiety. It may also help if you have abdominal cramps from heavy menstruation.

Coming in:

1. Cover your back and feet with a blanket or shawl.
2. 'Retreat from the world' by pulling the blanket over your head to create a 'cave' that feels cosy, calm, quiet and safe.

Caution: If you feel claustrophobic, remove the blanket.

Coming out:

1. Remove the blanket from your head and sit up kneeling in hero pose (virasana) for a few breaths.

QUEEN RECLINED SUPPORTED COBBLER'S POSE (RANI SALAMBA SUPTA BADDHA KONASANA)

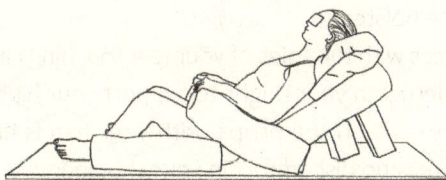

QUEEN RECLINED SUPPORTED COBBLER'S POSE (RANI SALAMBA SUPTA BADDHA KONASANA)

Benefits: This pose may relieve abdominal muscle cramps caused by menstruation and may feel cooling and calming for hot flushes. It also encourages a sense of physical and emotional opening, an attitude of relaxing and letting go, which is important in perimenopause. Please remember, though, that this is a supported relaxation pose and *not* a yin stretch. The aim is not to achieve a deep muscle stretch; the aim is to support your body in a position of ease (sattva).

Inflammation in menopause can affect your joints and connective tissues (including frozen shoulder, hips, lumbar spine, sacroiliac joint and knees). Treat yourself like a queen using as many props (cushions, pillows, bolsters, etc.) as you have available. Pay special attention to supporting your head and neck with a folded blanket. This 'head nest' stops it from rolling to the side so you can fully relax.

Before you settle into this pose, set a timer for 15 minutes so that your mind is not worrying about the time. (It takes a minimum of 10 minutes to fully relax your nervous system.)

Props: 1–2 bolsters or 2 firm pillows; 1–2 yoga bricks, 2–4 yoga blocks or cushions; 2–4 blankets. Optional: eye bag or mask, blanket to fold over body.

1. Place the bolster(s) or 2 firm pillows lengthways on your mat (or bed).
2. Elevate the top end with a yoga block, bricks or cushion underneath and adjust to a comfortable height.
3. Fold one blanket into a rectangle shape and lay it along the bolster, covering the lower end. This is to support the curve in your lower back.
4. Place props on either side of your mat to support your knees, hips and forearms. Fold a blanket at the top of your bolster to support your neck and head.

Coming in:

1. Sit your tailbone on the lower part of the blanket, and then lay your spine along the bolster.
2. Open your knees with the soles of your feet touching each other. Squish the props underneath your thighs to support your hips.
3. Rest your forearms on the props, with your hands higher than your elbows so there is no discomfort in your shoulders.
4. Fold the blanket under your neck and head so that your forehead is higher than your chin.
5. Option to place an eye bag or mask over your eyes or forehead to soften the light and allow your eyes to rest.

Tip: If your mind is active and you find it difficult to settle, listen to one of the yoga nidra recordings. If you are having hot flushes, repeat the hot flush wave affirmation in your mind as you practise ocean breath.

Modification for menstrual bleeding: If this wide knee pose causes menstrual flooding, you can either reduce the 'hip opening' by adding more props to support under your legs, or swap for a restorative side-lying pose (side lying savasana).

Modification for trauma and vulnerability: Place a rectangular folded blanket along the centre of your body and pelvis and cover your feet. The blanket weight can feel calming and comforting.

Coming out:

1. Use your hands to assist your legs up and allow your knees to touch, separating the feet wide. This is a gentle counterpose for the hips.
2. After a few breaths, sway your knees side to side gently (windshield wiper twist pose (supta parivrtta sucirandhrasana)), and roll over on to one side of your body to slowly come up to a seated position.

RESTORATIVE LEGS UP THE WALL POSE (VIPARITA KARANI)

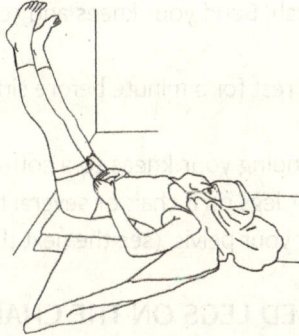

RESTORATIVE LEGS UP THE WALL POSE (VIPARITA KARANI), WITH BLANKET COCOON

Benefits: This inverted pose slows the heart rate and breathing pace down so it can feel mentally calming. The blanket cocoon around your head and neck is a form of sense withdrawal (pratyhara), so it may calm your mind and reduce anxiety and overwhelm by softening sounds and light. If you practise this pose at night with your legs up the wall behind your bed, it may help you drift off to sleep, so it could help with insomnia. Practise this pose during the day if you feel fatigued – it can help refresh your energy.

Props: 1 cushion or pillow; 1–2 blankets; 1 yoga strap or belt; optional eye bag or mask.

Coming in:

1. Place your mat up against a wall and open a large blanket over it. Place a cushion or pillow up against the wall.
2. Roll onto your back, so your pelvis is supported by the cushion and your legs are resting against the wall. Option to bind your legs together using a strap around your thighs.
3. Reach your arms overhead and drag the top of the blanket onto and around your head, pressing the material around your ears and neck. Option to cover your eyes with part of the blanket (like a hood) or place an eye bag onto your eyes or forehead.
4. Stay in the pose for 10 minutes during the daytime to restore energy if feeling fatigued. At night, stay as long as it takes to feel sleepy.

Coming out:

1. Be careful not to rush. Bend your knees and remove the strap or belt (if using).
2. Roll to one side and rest for a minute before sitting up.

Modify this pose by bending your knees to a softer 90-degree angle and resting the back on your legs on a chair or several bolsters, with a cushion or folded blanket under your pelvis. (see the next three restorative poses).

RESTORATIVE RAISED LEGS ON THE CHAIR (MODIFIED VIPARITA KARANI)

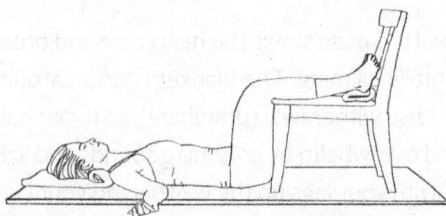

RESTORATIVE RAISED LEGS ON THE CHAIR (MODIFIED VIPARITA KARANI)

Benefits: Refreshes fatigue, reduces stress, may ease digestive issues. You can stay longer in this pose because it is less likely to cause leg numbing or discomfort.

Props: 2-3 blankets or pillows.

1. Bring your mat to a chair. (Alternatively, use a sofa or coffee table, and you can practise this pose on your bed with your legs supported by pillows.)
2. Fully open out a blanket on the mat so that it is flat and has no wrinkles. This is for warmth and lower back comfort.
3. Lower yourself sideways to the mat so that your pelvis is close to the chair. Option to rest your pelvis on a cushion (but not a bolster because it is too high).
4. Rest your legs onto a chair (sofa or bed) with your knees bent. If the chair edge is too hard, place a blanket over the edge. Make sure the backs of your knees are supported by folding a blanket over the edge for comfort.

5. Fold another blanket under your head and neck for support. Place your hands on your abdomen, out to the side or wrap your hands with the extra blanket for warmth. Option to place a weighted eye bag on your forehead or eyes, or a scarf if you wear contact lenses.

6. Stay in the pose for 15–20 minutes.

Coming out:

1. Be careful not to rush. Bend your knees.

2. Roll to one side and rest for a minute before sitting up.

Modification if you feel agitated or too hot: The sense withdrawal version of this pose involves the blanket tucked around your head and into your shoulders to cut out external sounds and stimulation. Remove the blanket, but stay in the pose with legs raised.

RESTORATIVE SHOULDER STAND (SALAMBA SARVANGASANA), WITH CHAIR AND BLANKETS

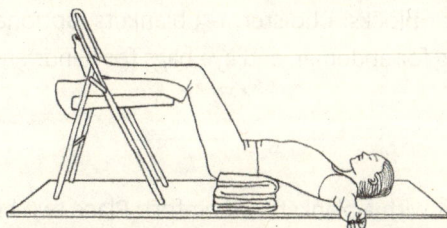

RESTORATIVE SHOULDER STAND (SALAMBA SARVANGASANA), WITH CHAIR AND BLANKETS

Benefits: This inversion lifts your hips higher with two blankets, but your legs are still supported by the chair so you are less likely to experience numbness, and you gain more benefits of an inversion, while allowing you to stay in the pose for 5–10 minutes.

Props: 3 or more blankets.

Coming in:

1. Place two or more folded blankets under your pelvis at a height that is comfortable for you.

2. Soften the edge of the chair with another blanket to support the back of your knees.

Coming out:

1. Lift your hips to remove the blankets and roll over to your side.

STONEHENGE RELAXATION POSE (MODIFIED SAVASANA)

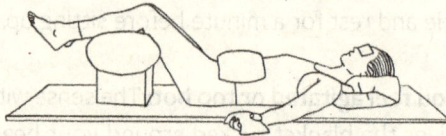

STONEHENGE RELAXATION POSE (MODIFIED SAVASANA)

Benefits: Refreshes fatigue, reduces stress, may ease digestive issues. You can stay longer in this pose than legs up a wall, because it is less likely to cause leg numbing or discomfort.

Props: 2 bricks or blocks; 1 bolster; 1–3 blankets; optional extra blanket, weighted sandbag for abdomen and eye bags for hands and eyes.

Coming in:

1. Cover the mat with a blanket for comfort. Place two bricks at the bottom of the mat and balance a bolster on the bricks to create a bridge or Stonehenge-type structure.
2. Lie down and support your neck and head with a pillow or folded blanket.
3. Rest the back of your knees on the bolster.

Options:

◎ Rest the back of your ankles on a smaller bolster or a rolled-up blanket.
◎ Place a weighted eye bag on your forehead or eyes to calm your mind. Alternatively, use a scarf to simply block out the light.
◎ Place a weighted sandbag on your abdomen for a sense of grounding.
◎ Support the back of your wrists with an eye bag or other prop (to relax your arms and shoulders), or place eye bags in the palms of your hands for a sense of grounding.

Coming out:

1. If you have an eye bag over your eyes or forehead, slowly slide it away from your skin so you don't disturb your nervous system.
2. Roll to your side and use your hands to sit upright.

RESTORATIVE SUPPORTED FISH POSE (SALAMBA MATSYASANA)

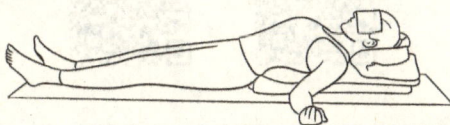

RESTORATIVE SUPPORTED FISH POSE (SALAMBA MATSYASANA)

Benefits: Gentle stretch across the chest and relaxes the shoulders. Restores energy, invites deeper breathing and encourages emotional sense of opening and positivity. This pose may subtly lift a low mood and lethargy.

Props: 1 blanket; optional extra pillow for neck and head; optional bolster, eye bag.

Coming in:

1. Fold a blanket into a large rectangle shape, then fan fold it into a narrower rectangle.
2. Place the blanket lengthways through the centre of your mat, then lay your spine down on the blanket.
3. Fold the top end of the blanket to support your head or add a pillow. Rest the back of your knees onto a bolster.
4. Open your arms and allow your shoulders to relax – this is a gentle chest-opening stretch.
5. Stay in the pose for 5–15 minutes.
6. Finish with a simple constructive rest pose (savasana) with your spine in a neutral position.

Modification for a fused tailbone: Sit on the end of the blanket. Lie back on the bolster, add a blanket or pillow to support the neck and head, place props under the legs and hips so there is no muscle strain, add an eye bag on the forehead or eyes (optional). To test: Focus on the breath, repeat the hot flush affirmation silently, or simply relax. Listen to guided meditation (optional). To exit: Use your hands to lift your knees together, slide the eye bag from your face, add a counterpose hip stretch, straighten your legs on the mat, open your eyes slowly, roll to the side and sit up.

Listen to these positive affirmations.

RESTORATIVE MOUNTAIN BROOK POSE

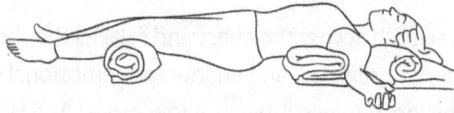

RESTORATIVE MOUNTAIN BROOK POSE

Props: 2 blankets; additional blanket or bolster.

Coming in:

1. Fold one blanket into a rectangle and lay it widthways along your mat. This is to support your shoulder blades and an open stretch across your chest.
2. Fold another blanket and place it at the top of your mat to support your head and neck. Support the back of your knees with either a bolster or rolled up blanket.
3. Stay for 5–10 minutes. If the chest stretch feels too intense, lower the blanket behind your shoulders or support your head with a block.

Coming out:

1. Bend your knees and roll over to one side of your body before sitting upright.

SUPPORTED WHEEL POSE (SALAMBA URDHVA DANURASANA), WITH BOLSTERS AND BLOCKS

Props: 1–3 bolsters; optional blocks or cushion.

1. Place 1–3 yoga bolsters on the mat widthways and lay your spine onto the bolsters. Depending on the bolster height, you may want to support your head and shoulders on blocks or a cushion.

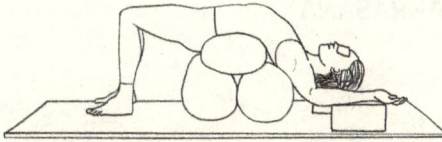

SUPPORTED WHEEL POSE (SALAMBA URDHVA
DANURASANA), WITH BOLSTERS AND BRICKS

RESTORATIVE FRONT-LYING PIGEON POSE (SALAMBA KAPOTASANA), WITH BOLSTER

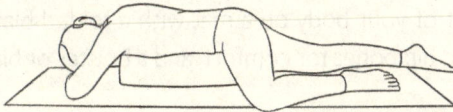

RESTORATIVE FRONT-LYING PIGEON POSE (SALAMBA KAPOTASANA), WITH BOLSTER

Benefits: May ease menstrual cramps, bloating and digestive issues. Downward facing poses can feel calming and grounding.

Props: 1 bolster; optional blanket.

Coming in:

1. Lay the front of your body over a bolster with one leg straight and one leg bent to the side.
2. Rest your forehead on your hands. Option to cover your back and head with a blanket.
3. Stay for 5 minutes then bend the other leg for 5 minutes.

Coming out:

1. Sit up and straddle the bolster for 5–10 rounds of breath.

Caution: If this causes abdominal discomfort or acid reflux, *stop* and practise a supported corpse pose (savasana) with your head higher than your stomach.

RESTORATIVE DOWNWARD FACING CORPSE POSE (ADVASANA), AKA CROCODILE POSE (SALAMBA MAKRASANA)

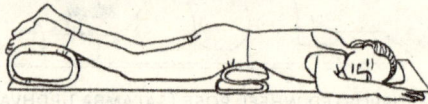

RESTORATIVE DOWNWARD FACING CORPSE POSE (ADVASANA),
AKA CROCODILE POSE (SALAMBA MAKRASANA)

Props: 1–2 blankets; 1 bolster.

1. Lay the front of your body on a mat with a folded blanket under your abdomen and hip bones for comfort, and a bolster or blanket to support your feet.
2. Turn your head to one side for a neck stretch, or rest your forehead on your hands.
3. Stay for 5–10 minutes (turn your head to both sides).

SIDE LYING RELAXATION POSE (MODIFIED SAVASANA)

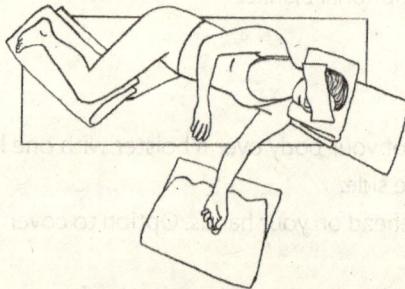

SIDE LYING RELAXATION POSE (MODIFIED SAVASANA),
WITH BLANKETS AND EYE PILLOW

Props: 3 blankets; optional: eye bag or scarf, bolster.

1. Lie down on your left side on a mat.
2. Place a folded blanket at the top of the mat to rest your head on. Use an eye bag or scarf if you want to cover your eyes. Place a folded blanket between your legs to support your thighs, knees and feet.
3. Rest your left hand on a blanket to relax your elbow and shoulder.
4. Press a long rolled-up blanket along your spine. Option to cover your body and head with a blanket.
5. Stay here for 10–15 minutes, then roll on to the right side of your body and adjust the props. Rest on your right side for 10–15 minutes.

Modification: Place a bolster at the front of your body and drape your right arm over or give it a hug; this may feel comforting.

Tip: Stay on one side of your body for 20 minutes if this is more comfortable for you.

Tip: Cover your back and head with a blanket, but keep a space open to breathe.

Caution: If you feel claustrophobic or anxious in this pose, exit whenever you choose.

SIDE LYING TWIST (SALAMBA SUPTA MATSEYANDRASANA), WITH BLANKETS

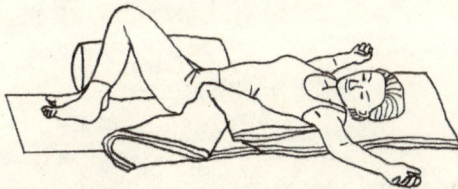

SIDE LYING TWIST (SALAMBA SUPTA MATSEYANDRASANA), WITH BLANKETS

Benefits: Aids digestion, supportive spinal twist, may ease menstrual cramps.

Props: 1 bolster or cushion; 2 large blankets; option: eye bag or scarf.

Coming in:

1. Place a bolster or cushion on the right side of your mat.
2. Place a folded-up blanket on your mat to support your back and shoulders. Roll up another blanket.
3. Lie down on your back, lower your bent legs to the right and rest them on the bolster.
4. Press the rolled-up blanket along your spine for warmth and support.
5. Stay in this supported twist for 5–10 minutes and then lower your bent legs to the left side of the mat, move the props and stay for 5–10 minutes.

Part Four

DAILY PRACTICES

EASTERN PHILOSOPHIES FOR MENOPAUSE

Slow down, tune in, bring in more yin.

Yang stress vs yin oestrogen

Indian Ayurveda and Traditional Chinese Medicine (TCM) view menopause as a natural life stage and hormonal transition requiring individualized holistic care. These Eastern healing systems offer a holistic approach that includes mind, body, emotions – and spirit or soul.

Indian Ayurveda suggests that stress disrupts the body's equilibrium, manifesting differently according to your individual constitution. The Ayurvedic concept of ida (the Moon, cool, calm feminine) and pingala (the Sun, heat, active, masculine) are similar to the TCM concept of hormones being yin (nourishing, cooling) and yang (active, warming) energies. Oestrogen is the most yin, while the stress hormones cortisol and adrenaline embody yang. You can visualize this balance as being like a see-saw. As your stress hormones go up, your oestrogen drops down. Optimal health hinges on a balance of both. In Ayurveda we call this balance sattva. In TCM it is depicted as the yin–yang symbol.[1]

In perimenopause your hormones fluctuate almost every day, so what you need to rebalance yourself will change each day. This is why a daily mindful yoga practice is so helpful in the perimenopause to menopause transition. Yoga helps you to slow down, tune in, bring in more yin – and whatever else you need to restore a daily sense of balance. Just 5–10 minutes of simple slow yoga breathing helps us to tune in to what we feel inside, where we feel it. This is your interoception.

Yoga and Buddhist philosophy helps us to understand that change is natural and beautiful, so we can relax instead of resisting. Resisting change is like trying to stop the flow of a river with your hand. Meditation gives us the mental clarity to see what we need, breathwork brings us back to a state of balance, and the yoga practice gives us mindful movement and poses that may ease physical symptoms.

MY mind: Psychological and cognitive symptoms

MY CLASS TO REDUCE STRESS

If you are feeling stressed, anxious or overwhelmed, use your breathing to find a sense of calm. This simple 5-minute practice uses abdominal breath with ocean sound to activate your body's relaxation response.

What you'll need:

- Yoga mat. For extra comfort, place a blanket on top of your mat.
- Optional pillow or folded blanket to support your head and neck during relaxation.
- No distractions. Set a timer with a calming sound (no loud alarms!). Let others know you need 5 minutes of quiet time. Taking care of yourself is a priority – a calmer you means everyone benefits!
- A peaceful environment. Enhance your practice with calming soundscapes like gentle ocean waves or a slow metronome to guide your breath.

5-minute practice

Abdominal breathing (adham pranayama) with ocean breath. Repeat for 5 minutes. You can either lie down or stay seated for this practice.

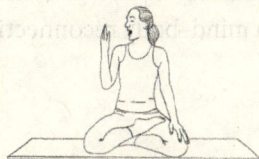

Afterwards, take a moment to notice how you feel. Do you feel a sense of calm washing over you? Are your muscles around your face and jaw starting to relax? Does your abdomen feel softer? You may notice gurgling sounds – that's your digestion working now you are relaxed.

15-minute practice

Start with abdominal breathing (adham pranayama) and then add the following:

Knees to chest pose (apanasana), moving slowly with your breath. The sensation of the foot on the mat can feel grounding. Repeat 10 times.

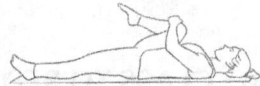

Windshield wiper twist pose (supta parivrtta sucirandhrasana), to relax your lower back. Repeat 8–10 times on both the left and right sides.

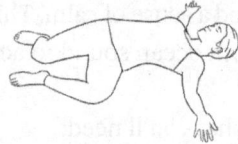

Roll on to the left side of the body for a few breaths, then bring yourself up gently to a seated position.

Oxytocin hug.

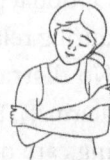

Repeat this positive affirmation 5–10 times:

'I am safe, I am well, I am cared for. I am peaceful and at ease. I can manage this, one breath at a time.'

Finish with either a seated meditation with a mudra (hand gesture) and a mantra, or choose the restorative pose suggested below (Stonehenge relaxation pose (modified savasana)) and listen to a yoga nidra to create a mind–body reconnection that brings you back to the present moment.

30-minute practice

Seated meditation with vata balancing (vayu mudra), 5 minutes.

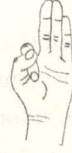

Practise abdominal breathing (adham pranayama) in and out of your nose. Try to slow down your exhalation for mental calm.

Repeat the 'I am that' (so-ham mantra) (or choose another mantra or affirmation that resonates with you). Observe your breath, noticing its rhythm and depth.

Stonehenge relaxation pose (modified savasana). Stay here for 20 minutes. You can listen to calming music during this pose.

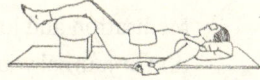

Watch these videos on reducing stress.[*]

BEYOND YOGA: TECHNIQUES FOR MENOPAUSE STRESS REDUCTION

- Acupressure: Apply pressure to points between the thumb and index finger, or with your thumb in the centre of your palm.
- Self-massage (abhyanga): Massage yourself with or without oil (add an oxytocin hug afterwards).
- EFT (emotional freedom techniques) tapping: Apply pressure on the hand muscle between your thumb and first finger.
- Spend time in Nature: Immerse yourself in the calmness of Nature (forest bathing, walks).
- Cold water therapy: Take cold plunges, showers or swims (best with friends).
- Earthing: Walk barefoot on grass.

[*] https://www.youtube.com/playlist?list=PLJ-mltZchfBB9d6nOWWnOCaYHP4aQDOWC

- Exercise.
- Sleep: Prioritize sleep and relaxation.
- Cognitive behavioural therapy (CBT): Helps you to observe your behaviour in stressful situations and develop new coping strategies. It focuses on the links between physical symptoms, thoughts, feelings and behaviour. The way we *think* about symptoms in certain situations tends to affect how we *feel* and what we *do*, and these reactions can in turn increase the intensity of bodily reactions. Using a journal can be a good place to start looking at your patterns of anxiety and stress, understanding what your triggers are, and how you can manage these emotions.
- Meditation and journaling prompts: Practise a gratitude meditation or journal your thoughts and feelings to gain insight into what is triggering your stress. In menopause your hormone fluctuations may be triggering anxiety, so notice where this occurs in your menstrual cycle. You may also be more sensitive to stimulants such as caffeine and even sugar, which means even one cup of coffee could trigger anxiety and heart palpitations. Write down what you eat and drink to help make these connections. Write down whether your stressful feelings are linked to feeling tired, lack of sleep or hunger. Or maybe you are too busy, overloading yourself with work or other responsibilities when you need to rest, do less and reduce stress. What are the absolute priorities? What could wait until another day? Instead of juggling plates, who could you delegate that task to? There are no prizes for being superwoman, and pushing through will just lead to burnout and fatigue.

Movement

The fight and flight response stores adrenaline and cortisol in your body, like a tightly wound coil, ready to be released to escape danger. But if the stress is in your head and you are stuck sitting at a computer, then you won't have any way to release that tension. Exercise, even walking, can help your body release these hormones and relax (see Part Two: Health and Wellbeing).

- Swimming: Gentle on joints; breathing deeply during swimming helps calm the nervous system and cold water is also good for cooling hot flushes.

- Aerobic exercise: Promotes deep breathing and releases stress hormones.
- Strength training: Maintains muscle mass and bone strength.
- Pilates: Improves core strength and helps with post-injury recovery.
- Moderate exercise: Avoid high-intensity classes or long gym sessions (this may cause fatigue and injury) and prioritize short bursts of activity – 5, 15 or 20 minutes.

Lifestyle

- Reduce caffeine intake: Limit caffeine or have it only in the morning.
- Blood sugar management: Eat regular meals and avoid blood sugar spikes/crashes.
- Nutrition: Focus on whole foods and protein and reduce processed foods and sugars. Avoid fasting.
- Social connection: Maintain social interactions to boost oxytocin (the bonding hormone).
- MY toolkit: Choose techniques that resonate with you and create a personalized stress reduction routine.

MY CLASS FOR ANXIETY

Stress is a general umbrella term, but we can hone it down to specific symptoms in order to help you define how you are feeling.

Anxiety is a form of mental stress caused by thinking into the future and worrying about events that have not yet happened. We may feel anxious for very good reasons, but in the menopause, the brain rewiring described by Dr Lisa Mosconi in her book *The Menopause Brain* may cause us to forward-project and fixate on the future in a way that is unhelpful. After all, the future is unknown.

Anyone, like me, who has experienced menopause anxiety will know how these thoughts can wake us up at night, overwhelm us during the day, and may even lead to heart palpitations and panic attacks. These are all known as vasomotor symptoms and are a real side effect of fluctuating and declining oestrogen, as well as the calming hormone progesterone.

Here are some daily practices that you can use to alleviate anxious thoughts. There is an overlap with 'MY class to reduce stress', but I have simplified the content and repeated movements because when we are anxious, we don't want a complicated practice.

Perimenopause, the season of Autumn and letting go

In Menopause Yoga, we associate perimenopause with Autumn (the Fall) because it is a season of change and transition that may include turbulence. One day the weather is hot and sunny and the next day it is wet and windy. The menopause is sometimes called 'The Change', and our hormones, moods, energy and symptoms can switch daily. These unpredictable fluctuations can swing from hot flushes to rage, anxiety to fatigue, rampant sexual drive and then low libido. Like a leaf falling from the tree, the perimenopause can make you feel ungrounded, blown about by the wind, anxious and unsure where you will land. It can feel like you are out of control and afraid of what is on the other side of menopause.

But there is also beauty in change: the colour of the leaves changes from green to red, gold and russet brown. There is wisdom in Nature. Autumn is a necessary season for letting go of what no longer supports the tree, especially as it needs to conserve energy through the winter. Our body is naturally letting go of the hormones needed for reproductivity. Would you feel less anxious if you chose to view your perimenopause positively as an opportunity to prioritize what really matters to you now? Could you let go of what no longer supports you physically, emotionally, practically? Like the tree releasing its leaves so it can conserve energy in its roots, you need to conserve your energy through the winter of your coming menopause. Letting go is a way to feel more in control. Reframe your perimenopause as a rite of passage, a necessary transition before you step into the next stage of your life – your Second Spring.

What you'll need:

- Yoga mat
- Block or weighted eye bag
- Blanket
- Bolster
- Cloth or scarf
- Listen to this simple breathing affirmation to calm anxiety.

5-minute practice

Seated meditation: Mind meets the breath (with a block or weighted eye bag on the crown of your head). Sit comfortably upright, with your knees level with, or lower than, your hips. Sit up onto a block or a cushion if required.

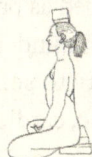

15-minute practice

Cat-cow-child's pose (marjaryasana-bitilasana-balasana) flow, for 8–10 rounds.

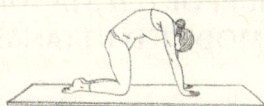

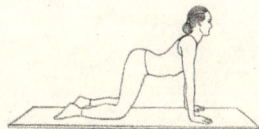

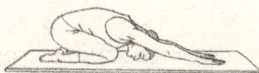

Child's pose (balasana), resting forehead on hands, fists or yoga block. Stay for 4–8 breaths.

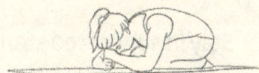

Downward facing dog pose (adho mukha svanasana). Stay for 4–8 breaths (30–60 seconds).

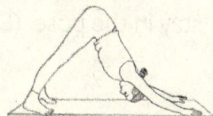

30-minute practice

End with a restorative supported child's pose (salamba balasana) with raised bolster and option to 'retreat from the world' with a blanket covering your back and head. Stay for 10 minutes (turn your head to the other side after 5 minutes).

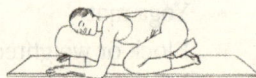

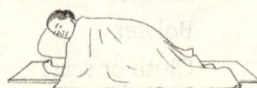

Watch these videos for reducing anxiety parts 1, 2 and 3.[*]

The power of mind–body connection is indisputable and is widely used as part of a mindfulness practice. In medical terms this mind–body connection is called 'interoception', the ability to sense the internal state of your body using the nervous, endocrine, cardiorespiratory and gastrointestinal systems.

Here are some additional poses and practices that you may like to try. It's important to find the tools and techniques that work best for you.

SUPPORTED STANDING FORWARD FOLD (MODIFIED UTTANASANA)

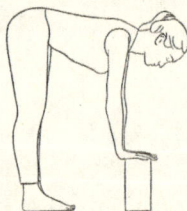

SUPPORTED STANDING FORWARD FOLD (MODIFIED UTTANASANA), WITH BRICKS

1. Stay in supported standing forward fold for 8–10 breaths. Use props such as an upturned bolster, bricks or a chair and bend your knees to help you stay in the pose. (See 'Using props for modifications'.)

---

* https://www.youtube.com/playlist?list=PLJ-mltZchfBB9d6nOWWnOCaYHP4aQDOWC

SUPPORTED SEATED FORWARD FOLD
(MODIFIED PASCHIMOTTANASANA)

1. Stay in supported seated forward fold for 8–10 breaths.

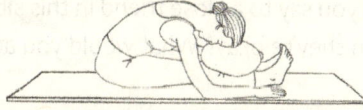

SUPPORTED SEATED FORWARD FOLD (MODIFIED
PASCHIMOTTANASANA), WITH BOLSTER

HEAD WRAPPING

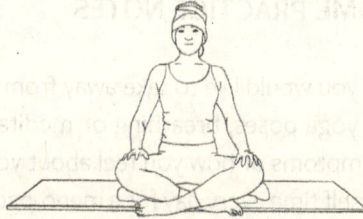

SEATED HEAD WRAPPING

Wrapping a cloth or scarf around your head has a calming effect on your mind and nervous system. It works in a similar way to the gentle pressure we place on the crown chakra and third eye marma point, with the added benefit of feeling held and contained. There are several marma or acupressure points on the head that are believed to help calm the mind. One of these is located at the space between your eyebrows (third eye centre), another one is in the middle of your forehead, and there is one on the crown or top of your head.

YOGA NIDRA FOR EASING ANXIETY

1. Listen to this nidra in 'Yoga basics'.
2. Repeat the loving-kindness meditation (metta bhavana).
3. Breathe. Practise ocean breath (ujjayi pranayama) through the nose. Sit with a straight back, hands on thighs. Close your eyes.
4. Take 10 rounds of breath, lengthening your inhalation and exhalation for as long as you feel comfortable.

5. Objectively question: Are your thoughts and fears 'catastrophizing'? In other words, thinking the worst outcome? What is the evidence to support your view of a situation? Are you being overly negative? Are you underestimating your ability to cope? Have you managed similar situations before? When you faced this situation, and you managed it well? What would you say to a close friend in this situation? How would you reassure them they're okay? What would you advise them to do?

Remember: Anxious/stressful thoughts are *not facts* – they are just thoughts, they are one viewpoint, usually exaggerated/catastrophized in the heat of your emotion.

Watch or listen to this meditation for calming your mind.

JOURNALING/HOME PRACTICE NOTES

1. Write down what you would like to take away from this practice today.
2. Did any of these yoga poses, breathing or meditation feel helpful in managing your symptoms or how you feel about your menopause?
3. Can you give yourself time every day for a meno-*pause* – more time and space to rest in daily life? This can be as little as 15 minutes or longer, but you will benefit more if you include it every day.
4. How would it feel to do less in your daily life? What is absolutely necessary for you to do, and what could you drop to avoid overloading your day? What are your priorities?
5. What activities make you feel calmer? Yoga, walking in Nature, swimming, calling a friend, reading a book, rest?

MY CLASS FOR OVERWHELM

I'd felt stressed in the past, who hasn't? I was in a senior role at work and always got things done. But when perimenopause hit, I felt overwhelmed by the simplest task. I just wanted to hide away from the world. I couldn't work, I couldn't go out, I couldn't even make decisions about food shopping. Yoga really helped me. (Anon.)

Overwhelm is a form of anxiety that may also be accompanied by heart palpitations or a panic attack. Although it is not a medical term, it perfectly describes the feeling of fear and inaction. Remember, the brain rewiring that starts at perimenopause makes it harder for us to manage stress. But your primitive stress response is not just isolated to fight and flight; there is also the freeze response. Staying still and barely breathing to become 'invisible' to predators may have saved our ancestors, and you may have unconsciously used this tactic if caught in the middle of conflict at home or work. But in your menopause, the freeze response can become so debilitating you can't function. So how can you become unstuck?

The quickest way to unfreeze is to deepen your breathing and use mind–body connection techniques. To bring yourself down from that sense of panic, it helps to come into the present moment through the power of touch. There are many techniques, including emotional freedom techniques (EFT), which involve tapping meridian lines on your body with the tips of your fingers. Other simple techniques include self-massage and touching specific parts of your body and naming them.

Here is a simple 5-minute practice for overwhelm, using self-touch and massage.

5-minute practice

Start with simple abdominal breathing (adham pranayama), either lying down or seated.

Use your hands to touch or gently massage your face, naming the parts of your face one by one: nose, eyelids, forehead, crown of head, back of head, ears, jaw, cheeks, lips, chin, neck.

Touch your chest, collarbone, shoulders, arms, elbows, wrists, hands, fingers – naming each part. Continue through the front of your body touching your ribs, abdomen, hips, thighs, knees, ankles and feet, then either up the inside or back of your legs, and the back of your body.

Return to your head again and end with one hand resting on your heart and the other on your abdomen for a sense of anchoring.

Repeat a positive affirmation that works for you. For example: 'I am safe, I am grounded, I am here.'

Give yourself an oxytocin hug.

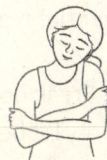

Watch this Ocean breath video for easing overwhelm.[*]

Here are some other techniques that you may find helpful. I've given you positive affirmations, a CBT exercise and 'My daily priority list' to help you prioritize and plan. When we panic, we cannot think clearly and may freeze with indecision. Changing your perspective on an overwhelming situation and breaking a big job into small tasks can help you to become unstuck.

Listen to these positive affirmations. How do they make you feel?

Positive affirmations:

I breathe in joy,
I breathe out fear.

I breathe in calm,
I breathe out worry.

Cognitive behavioural therapy for overwhelm

Remind yourself of a time when you have felt overwhelmed in the past and how you coped. What techniques did you use, what did you do to feel able to cope? Could you use those same techniques or positive thoughts in your current situation? Or could you adapt them? You have successfully done this in the past, so remind yourself:

> I can do *this*,
> I *can* do this,
> I can do this,
> One *breath* at a time/One *step* at a time.

Kindness and self-compassion are key to feeling calmer.

Then we can use CBT to ask ourselves, what are we are afraid of? Is there a fear of failing, not completing a task to a standard of perfection? How would it feel to adequately complete the task? What is the priority? How essential really is this task?

Journal: Break down the task in front of you into smaller chunks (see 'My daily priority list below'). Smaller chunks are easier to achieve. If we complete

---

* https://www.youtube.com/playlist?list=PLJ-mltZchfBB9d6nOWWnOCaYHP4aQDOWC

one step or chunk of the task, the others will feel more manageable. In yoga, we take a *krama* approach to life on and off the mat. It means wise progression, or one step at a time.

'To do' lists

I used to have 10 things on my 'To do' list every day. Did I complete them all? Never, so they just rolled over to the next day and a new list.

Now in my postmenopause I advise you to join me in a radical act of realism: only put five things on your list and make two of them feeding yourself nourishing food and gentle exercise, preferably outdoors in Nature, and with friends. The other three tasks can be work- or home-related – but see if you can add a simple daily dose of joy such as singing or dancing as you do your household chores, or listen to your favourite music, or a podcast, while shopping or commuting to work. Stroking a pet animal and hugging a loved one can release oxytocin. The possibilities are endless. Find some joy in the tasks themselves or do them with a friend. With less on your list you will always succeed – and that feeling of success reduces stress and helps you rest.

For 'My daily priority list', tick when each task is completed.

My daily priority list

Tick	Task	What, when, where, why
1	Movement Exercise with friends/in Nature	
2	Nourishment Healthy foods that feed my bones, brain, muscles and a happy gut	
3	Home/house Cleaning, shopping, cooking, organizing	
4	Commitments Prioritize a work or volunteering task that needs to be started or completed today	
5	Commitments [please add your own here]	

MY CLASS FOR BRAIN FOG

Brain fog may trigger a sense of overwhelm because simple tasks at work or home feel impossible. Some people describe brain fog as not being able to connect their thoughts, as if their cognitive function feels slow, and you may have temporary lapses in your short-term memory retrieval, forgetting the name of your child or the name of a street. I have done this many times! The good news is that brain fog can clear, and the short-term memory lapse is exactly that – short term. Usually, the word comes back to you later when you relax. Dr Lisa Mosconi's research and brain scan images show that the rewiring of your brain in perimenopause to menopause is completed by postmenopause, so your memory and cognitive function can bounce back. In fact, she says your brain deliberately lets go of functions it no longer needs (such as how to lactate and breastfeed) and gets an 'upgrade' so it becomes 'leaner' and keener in postmenopause.[2]

Sometimes our foggy head is the result of a broken night's sleep due to night sweats or trips to the bathroom. So you may also experience a daytime fatigue. Choose either the following energizing uplifting practice ('Clearing brain fog') to wake you up and clear cognitive brain fog or the afternoon meno-*pause* physical fatigue practice ('MY morning class for fatigue' and 'MY afternoon class for fatigue') to restore depleted energy.

Clearing brain fog

Here are three short 5-minute breathing practices that can help clear brain fog and may give you an energy boost. Try them all and choose one that works for you. Put it in your toolkit to use whenever you feel a lack of mental focus. You will need a yoga mat or a comfortable chair or place to sit and a yoga strap.

5-minute practice

Slow bellows breath (modified slow kapalabhati breathing).

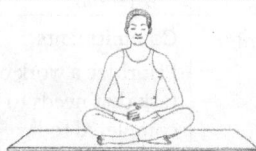

5-minute practice

Strap breathing (parts 1, 2, 3). Observe how you feel, the quality of your breathing, and whether your mind feels clearer or your body feels more energized.

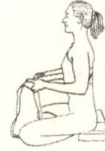

5-minute practice

Breath of joy (either seated or standing). Repeat for 10 rounds.

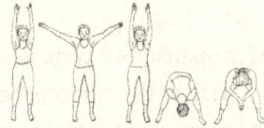

Watch this video on clearing brain fog.[*]

MY emotions: Mood swings

Menopause is a time when emotions from the previous part of our lives can rise to the surface. Some of these emotions may have been submerged for some time, waiting to be processed. They can get stuck in the body and manifest as physical pain. You may feel a sense of grief or loss as you prepare for the next stage of your life. You may not feel ready to change, let go of your menstrual cycle or the possibility of having children – if you wanted them. There may also be bereavement of parents, the end of a marriage or relationship, or maybe you feel a loss from leaving a job and career that you once loved.

MY CLASS FOR RELEASING OUR EMOTIONAL ARMOUR

Yoga poses and movements that stretch the muscles around your rib cage can help you breathe more deeply and release physical and emotional tension, according to yoga teacher and author Max Strom.[3]

5-minute practice

Strap breathing (parts 1, 2, 3).

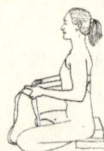

Deep breathing techniques may cause emotions to come to the surface. You may feel tearful or angry. Give yourself time and space after this practice. If any emotions arise that you feel unable to manage on your own, please seek professional counselling support. This may be an opportunity to process the past in a healthy way to help you move on to your future.

MY CLASS FOR MENORAGE AND IRRITABILITY

Menorage feels like a surge of energy that consumes me and in that flare of rage I feel 100 per cent justified for being angry. It is like a whole lifetime of inequality and injustice explodes. Afterwards I feel guilty and exhausted like I'm burnt out. (Rachel)*

Menopause rage (menorage) is a modern phrase for the surge in irritability and anger that you may feel in the menopause. This emotion may suddenly surge from 0–100 in an instant, and be so forceful that it takes you, and others, by surprise. In the past this rage has been negatively labelled 'hysteria' or 'insanity'. These labels are deep-seated in our history and culture and are linked to the caricature of menopausal women as mad or as witches, not easily tamed, talking back to men and behaving in a way that was socially unacceptable for women. A more positive phrase is 'power surges', and in Traditional Chinese Medicine (TCM) they are viewed as a sign of Second Spring, when you step into your power.

These emotions are partly triggered by the hormonal rewiring of our brain that affects our ability to produce the happy calming hormones serotonin, noradrenaline, oxytocin and dopamine that help us manage stress. These emotions may have been simmering for a long time until the point of exhaustion and overwhelm from multitasking for work, friends and family, and long-term lack of sleep causing allostatic overload. Imagine your energetic resources are a pot of soup you have been dishing out to feed and nourish others for years, so when you reach perimenopause there is nothing left for you. You are literally scraping the bottom of the pot and wondering why you feel so depleted, stressed and angry. Isn't it about time somebody else nourished you with soup and self-care?

Did you know that dentists are often the first people to notice you are in perimenopause because your gums may recede and you may

---

* A pseudonym has been used here to protect anonymity.

start to clench your teeth at night? This is the anxiety dreams and past memories resurfacing. You may need a tooth guard.

Men do not own anger, women do not own love. We are all capable of all of these human emotions. We are not mad or bad. The next time you feel angry or irritable, say yourself: 'How very human of me. I am feeling an emotion.' (Petra Coveney)

Rebecca Traister[4] highlights the disparity in attitudes towards men's anger, which is viewed as normal, and women's anger, which is viewed as unacceptable. Perhaps you too have felt a sense unfairness about the lack of a role for older women in society that may makes you feel unfulfilled and undervalued? Oestrogen is like a veil covering our eyes. As our oestrogen declines, the veil lifts and we may see clearly for the first time the gender injustice.

Do you explode or implode?

Have you noticed how you feel an energy surge when you are irritable? Like a pot of boiling water the heat and energy needs to go somewhere. If we cover the pot, we are likely to 'flip our lid' and explode with emotion. Exploding with anger may hurt people we care for and fail to communicate our feelings because people shut their ears when we shout. But imploding and suppressing that emotion could harm you, leading longer term to a low mood and depression, or physical side effects such as headaches and problems with digestion and elimination.

These Menopause Yoga tools and short practices are designed to help you channel that energy and heated emotions in a constructive way so that you don't flip your lid or internally combust. You may be justified in feeling angry or outraged, but if you can step back from the brink, take a few focused breaths, it may help you to communicate more effectively what you need people to hear. And you'll feel more in control.

This short class helps to release unexpressed emotion that we may hold tightly in our jaw and hips with a stretch to stimulate a physical yawn. Have you ever noticed how relaxed you feel after yawning? This is because it stimulates your vagal nerve, which helps you switch from stress to rest, which is why we yawn before sleeping. The restorative pose at the end is to restore your energy after feeling burnt-out emotion. Remember: you are not good or bad – these are just emotions. Practise this regularly and it can help prevent the build-up of anger; it's a healthy pressure valve release.

Note: If you are a person who implodes (turns the emotion inwards on yourself) you may be feeling angry and depressed, so try the 'MY class for low mood' to see if this helps.

Menopause rage

Choose one of these three breathing techniques and practise 3 rounds of 10 breaths. Then breathe naturally and notice how you feel.

5-minute practice

Lion's breath (simhasana pranayama). Repeat for 4–8 breaths.

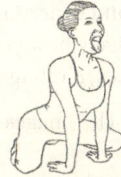

Hissing breath (sitkari pranayama). This breathing technique helps you let of steam, releasing rising tension. Repeat 3 x 10 rounds of breaths.

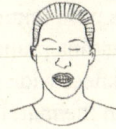

Blowing birthday candle breath. Visualize a birthday cake with candles – as many as your age. This is a celebration of you and the life you have lived so far, so you can make it the most delicious cake you like. Repeat 3 x 10 rounds of breaths.

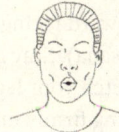

'My true self' (sa ta na ma mantra).

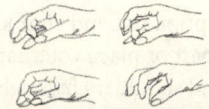

After your breathing practice, sit quietly and observe how you feel in your body, mind and emotions.

Journaling: Did any of these breathing techniques help you to simmer down from the heat of your menorage? Does your energy feel more balanced?

Are you more able to express your feelings calmly? Write down which of these breathing and meditation techniques worked for you. Next time you feel a surge of anger, ask yourself, how can I communicate these important feelings in a way that will be heard?

15-minute practice

Start with one of the breathing techniques, then continue with these poses.

Cat-cow (marjaryasana-bitilasana) flow with hip circles. Start with cat-cow-child's pose (marjaryasana-bitilasana-balasana) flow, then widen your knees apart and add in some hip and shoulder joint circles. Make these movements fluid and generous. Close your eyes and sense intuitively how your body wants to move. Repeat 10 times, circling clockwise and anticlockwise.

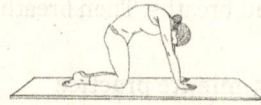

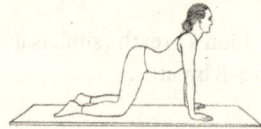

Note: The images do not show the hip circles.

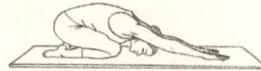

Lion's pose (simhasana) with lion's breath (simhasana pranayama). Sit on your heels with your knees wide apart and your hands in front of you on the mat. Practise lion's breath 4–8 times.

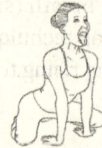

Downward facing dog pose (adho mukha svanasana). Stay for 4–8 breaths. Use this pose to stretch your legs and spine after kneeling. Pressing firmly into the floor can release physical tension in your muscles.

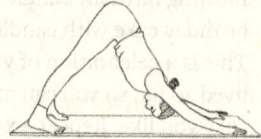

Option to bend your knees, step your feet wider apart or place your hands on bricks if your neck and shoulders feel tight.

Low crescent lunge pose (modified anjaneyasana) with cactus arms (bend your arms in a right angle shape aka cactus arms) (right leg)

Hold this pose for 4 breaths with the option to use lion's breath (simhasana pranayama) or one of the other menorage breathing techniques, e.g. hissing breath, blowing birthday candle breath.

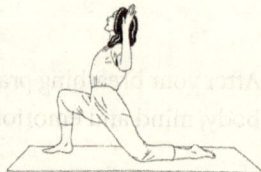

Lizard pose (utthan pristhasana), right leg, for 4–6 breaths.

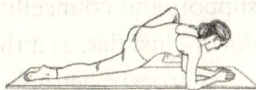

Side lunges (skandasana), 4–8 times, moving from side to side slowly. Use props to modify.

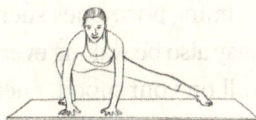

Child's pose (balasana) or downward facing dog pose (adho mukha svanasana), for 4–6 breaths.

Low crescent lunge pose (modified anjaneyasana) with cactus arms (left leg), for 4 breaths.

Lizard pose (utthan pristhasana), left leg, for 4–6 breaths.

Side lunges (skandasana), 4–8 times.

Child's pose (balasana), for 4–6 breaths. Rest your forehead on your hands or fists or a block to calm your mind.

30-minute practice

Restorative supported bridge pose (modified salamba setu bandhasana).

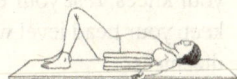

Downward facing corpse pose (advasana) aka crocodile pose (salamba makrasana).

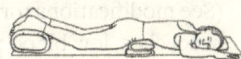

End with a relaxation pose (savasana) for 10 minutes.

Watch these videos to soothe menopause rage parts 1, 2 and 3.*

MY CLASS FOR LOW MOOD (ANHEDONIA)

Menopause low mood has a medical name and definition – anhedonia – which means loss of joy. This is distinct from other forms of clinical depression (for which you are advised to seek professional medical

* https://www.youtube.com/playlist?list=PLJ-mltZchfBB9d6nOWWnOCaYHP4aQDOWC

support and counselling). Anhedonia is when you feel neither up nor down – just flat, as if the sky is grey, day after day after day.

Low oestrogen affects your brain's ability to produce your happy and calming hormones such as dopamine, serotonin and noradrenaline. You may also be waking every night, so chronic insomnia and fatigue take their toll on your mood, energy and outlook on life. Everything seems better after a good night's sleep, doesn't it?

When we are feeling sad, tired, hopeless or maybe experiencing grief and loss of self-identity in our menopause, our posture slumps, our shoulders round and we draw physically and emotionally inward. In this position, it is impossible to breathe deeply or feel energetic and positive.

This is an energizing and uplifting class with dynamic 'heart opening' designed to shift stagnant (tamasic) energy and help lift a low mood. Hatha poses include and make space for your lungs to expand.

5-minute practice

Breath of joy. Repeat for 10 rounds and then bend your knees, rest your elbows on your thighs and keep your head level with your heart, to avoid dizziness.

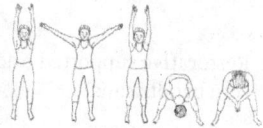

(See modifications for osteoporosis, hot flushes, headaches, low blood pressure and glaucoma on.)

15-minute practice

Sun salutation (surya namaskar), for 1 round.

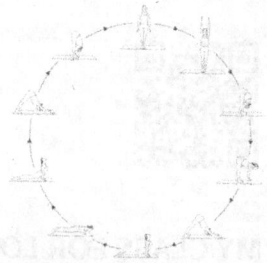

Plank pose (phalankasana), either high or knees on mat. Option to place your hands on bricks. Stay for 5–10 breaths.

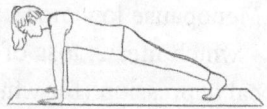

Downward facing dog pose (adho mukha svanasana), for 5 breaths.

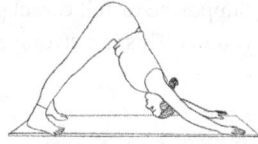

Locust pose (salabhasana). Lift chest, arms and legs for 2 rounds of 5 breaths. Option to place blanket under hip bones for comfort.

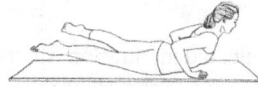

Child's pose (balasana), for 5 breaths.

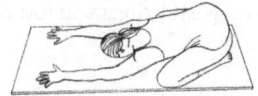

Downward facing dog pose (adho mukha svanasana), for 2–4 breaths.

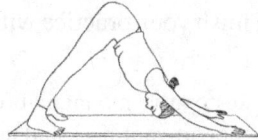

Mountain pose (tadasana), at the front of the mat, for 2–4 breaths.

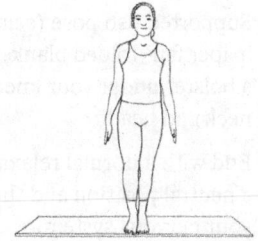

Chair pose (modified utkatasana), with a brick or block between the thighs.

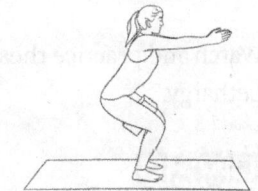

Meno-warrior chair pose squats (modified utkatasana), for 10 rounds.

Mountain pose (tadasana), eyes closed, for 2–4 breaths.

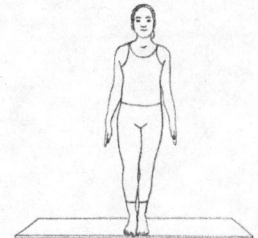

Supported or full camel pose (ustrasana), for 3 rounds. This is a strong energizing pose.

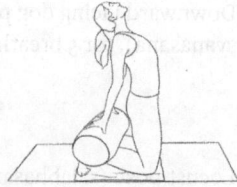

Seated meditation: sit comfortably with legs crossed, or in hero's pose for 5–10 breaths. Have the palms of your hands resting on your heart and focus on what brings you joy, or a gratitude meditation.

30-minute practice

Finish your practice with one of these restorative poses for 10 minutes.

Restorative mountain brook pose. Add props to support your neck and head for comfort.

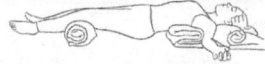

Supported fish pose (salamba matsyasana), with a 'paper fan'-folded blanket supporting your spine, a bolster under your knees and support for your neck and head.

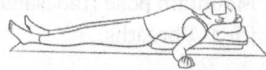

End with a normal relaxation pose (savasana) so that the spine can settle in a neutral position and the therapeutic effects of this practice can settle into your nervous system.

Watch and practice these videos for Breath of Joy, Lifting Low Mood and Lethargy.*

---

* https://www.youtube.com/playlist?list=PLJ-mltZchfBB9d6nOWWnOCaYHP4aQDOWC

MY body: Physical symptoms

MY CLASS FOR HOT FLUSHES AND NIGHT SWEATS

Hot flushes or flashes, a vasomotor symptom, are sudden feelings of intense heat, often accompanied by:

- Increased heart rate
- Skin redness
- Sweating.

Night sweats are hot flushes that occur during sleep, leading to waking up feeling hot and sweaty or cold and clammy. Anxiety, especially during night terrors, can worsen these symptoms.

Hot flushes and night sweats are caused by fluctuations in oestrogen levels affecting the hypothalamus, the brain region that controls body temperature. This sensitivity can trigger hot flushes and chills. Stressful thoughts can also trigger adrenaline release, mimicking hot flushes. Declining oestrogen may increase body-wide inflammation, contributing to hot flushes.

Symptoms can be managed by:

- Identifying and eliminating trigger foods such as caffeine, alcohol, spicy foods and sugar
- Increasing phytoestrogen-rich foods such as soy products, lentils and leafy greens (except for women with a history of breast cancer)
- Dressing in breathable, layered clothing made from natural fibres
- Keeping your environment cool and avoiding hot showers or rooms

- Developing a relaxation routine before bed to manage night sweats.

As a medical treatment, hormone replacement therapy (HRT) can help regulate hormones and reduce hot flushes. Discuss this option with your doctor, especially if you have a history of breast cancer, fibroids or endometriosis.

If night sweats disrupt your sleep, note down the time you wake up, what you ate/drank before bed, and any stimulants consumed (caffeine, screens, etc.). Late-night eating and stimulants can affect digestion and body temperature, leading to night sweats.

Night sweats can be managed by:

- Getting out of bed and cooling down
- Changing nightclothes and bedding
- Drinking water and avoiding digital screens before bed
- Ensuring proper airflow by keeping a window slightly open.

Certain herbal remedies may help (sage, black cohosh – although consult a doctor before use), aromatherapy (clary sage, fennel, peppermint) and phytoestrogen-rich foods can offer additional support. However, women with a history of breast cancer should avoid soy products.

Try these three cooling breath techniques and choose one that works best for you. Practise 3 rounds of 10 breaths. When you consciously change your breathing, it may cause you dryness in your mouth and throat. This is normal. Sip some room-temperature water before each breathing technique to moisten your mouth.

Cooling breath techniques

- Straw breath (kaki pranayama): Inhale slowly through pursed lips, exhale slowly.
- Smiling (or hissing) breath (sitkari pranayama): Inhale through sides of mouth, exhale slowly.
- Funnel breath: Curl tongue, inhale slowly through the narrowed space, exhale slowly.
- Modified funnel (curled tongue) breath (sitali pranayama): Option to lift chin as you breathe in through your curled tongue. Then hold your breath as you lower your chin down towards your chest, and exhale. This is the most effective cooling breath technique but can cause some

people to feel dizzy or nauseous. Stop if you feel unwell and breathe naturally. Sip some water.

15-minute practice

Abdominal breathing (adham pranayama) in constructive rest pose (savasana). Lay down on the mat with your knees bent and feet on the floor. Begin your three-part breathing into the abdomen, ribs and chest, with one hand on your abdomen and one hand on your chest.

Add ocean breath for 10 breaths. Visualize heat rising with the inhale, releasing with the exhale.

Hot flush wave. Silently repeat: 'This is just a hot flush, It will not last. I let it flow through me. The heat will pass.'

Knee and hip circles to stretch the hips and groin.

Windshield wiper twist pose (supta parivrtta sucirandhrasana).

Cat-cow (marjaryasana-bitilasana) flow. Slowly exhale out of your mouth with ocean breath.

Wide knee child's pose (balasana). Rest your forehead on a brick or block, arms extended forward, to allow heat to release.

30-minute practice

Finish your practice with this supported version of reclined cobbler's pose (salamba supta baddha konasana). This queen version uses lots of props to support your body in this hip and chest open pose, to help release physical heat and calm your nervous system, and give you a sense of emotional support.

Queen reclined supported cobbler's pose (salamba supta baddha konasana).

Journaling: Which of the breathing techniques felt cooler for you? Can you add this to 'MY toolkit' and try practising when you feel a hot flush? Write down what you eat, drink, do (including exercise, conversations and digital screen time). Do you notice any connections between what you consume and hot flushes or night sweats? These are your triggers. Could you reduce these in your daily life for a week and see if it helps?

Watch and practice these videos for cooling hot flushes.*

Cognitive behavioural therapy for hot flushes

Research by Myra Hunter and Melanie Smith[5] proved that slow, 'paced' breathing techniques and CBT were effective for women in clinical trials to help reduce the frequency of hot flushes, and they have been recommended by the British and International Menopause Societies. Paced breathing is the same as the slow abdominal breathing we use in yoga to reduce stress. The CBT techniques invite participants to change their negative thoughts to positive ones. This is similar to the 'think positive' (pratipaksha bhavana) philosophy in Patanjali's yoga sutras. These techniques help train our mind to respond calmly instead of reacting impulsively.

Hot flushes are steeped in social stigma, and sexual stereotyping may cause women in some cultures to feel embarrassed to sweat profusely in public. This stressful reaction to hot flushes can exacerbate them, making them hotter, last longer and become more frequent. The more we relax and accept these sensations, the faster they fade and decline over time.[6]

Read the imagined conversation below, and notice how a negative thought can escalate into worse symptoms:

Oh no, I can't cope.	*Let's see how well I can deal with this one, one flush at a time.*
Everyone is looking at me.	*I will notice my flushes more than other people; they may not notice.*
I am out of control.	*There are things I can do to take control.*
They will go on for ever.	*They will gradually reduce over time.*

Hot flushes may make you feel out of control of your own body and this can be frightening. Challenge your perception. Are your negative thoughts making your symptoms worse? Which voice makes you feel calmer or more in control? How does it feel to view hot flushes from a different perspective?

---

* https://www.youtube.com/playlist?list=PLJ-mltZchfBB9d6nOWWnOCaYHP4aQDOWC

Cold chills

Some people experience cold chills instead of hot flushes. The root cause is the same – your hypothalamus temperature gauge becomes over-sensitive – but instead of sending blood to the skin surface to release heat, your body may draw heat away from your extremities (hands and feet) towards your heart.

Try these simple yoga techniques to stimulate blood flow. Add ginger, turmeric and black pepper to your diet for circulation and include regular aerobic exercise 'snacks' to move your body.

5-minute practice

Slow, gentle bellows breath (slow kapalabhati breathing), 3 rounds of 10 breaths, pausing in between each round to check there is no dizziness.

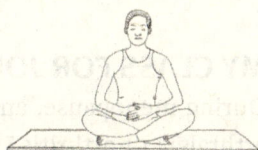

Breath of joy, for 10 rounds.

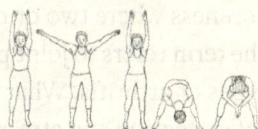

15-minute practice

Meno-warrior chair pose squats (modified utkatasana), 3 rounds of 10 squats with arm movements.

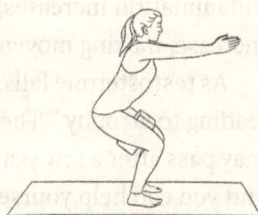

Goddess high squat pose (utkata konasana), with 10 small pulsing movements. Pulse up and down making small movements with your legs in a squat position.

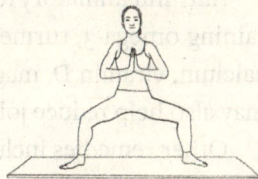

(See 'MY class for strength'.)

30-minute practice

Start with one of the breathing techniques (e.g., slow bellows breath (slow kapalabhati breathing) or breath of joy, and then add self-massage, stroking your body and limbs to stimulate blood flow. Option to add a warming aromatherapy oil. (See instructions for 'Self-massage (abhyanga) with oils'.)

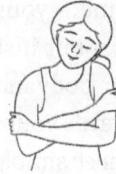

Watch this breathing technique for creating more heat in your body and boosting circulation.[*]

MY CLASS FOR JOINT AND MUSCLE PAIN

During menopause, an estimated 50 per cent of women experience arthralgia or arthritis.[7] Arthralgia is the medial term for joint pain or soreness where two or more bones meet. Arthritis isn't a single disease; the term refers to joint pain or joint disease, and there are more than 100 types of arthritis. What links arthralgia and most arthritic conditions is inflammation and stress.[8]

Joints have oestrogen receptors, which are affected by the loss of oestrogen in menopause, and arthralgia can affect your ability to exercise, leading to muscle loss and weight gain. When oestrogen levels drop and inflammation increases, the risk of osteoporosis and osteoarthritis can increase, making movement painful.

As testosterone falls, it becomes harder to maintain muscle strength, leading to atrophy.[**] The good news is that menopause-related arthralgia may pass after a few years when your hormone levels have settled down, and you can help yourself by living a healthy lifestyle.[9]

Anti-inflammatory foods can reduce symptoms, such as oily fish containing omega-3, turmeric, ginger, cinnamon and garlic. Foods rich in calcium, vitamin D, magnesium zinc, essential fatty acids and collagen may also help reduce joint pain.[10]

Other remedies include:

---

[*] https://www.youtube.com/playlist?list=PLJ-mltZchfBB9d6nOWWnOCaYHP4aQDOWC
[**] Ko J, Park YM. Menopause and the Loss of Skeletal Muscle Mass in Women. Iran J Public Health. 2021 Feb;50(2):413-414. doi: 10.18502/ijph.v50i2.5362. PMID: 33748008; PMCID: PMC7956097.

- Herbal: Liquorice, black cohosh, German chamomile, red clover, dandelion root
- Massage and essential oils: Clary sage, cypress, rosemary, lemongrass, lavender
- Supplements: Magnesium
- Complementary therapy: Acupuncture for the specific muscles and also for kidney balance to reduce dehydration in your tissues
- Exercise: Movement is good, especially swimming, and gentle, somatic yoga movement.

Joint mobilizing sequence (pawanmuktasana)

In yoga therapy we use a joint-freeing daily practice that can both help alleviate and prevent stiffness. The sequence in this book was inspired by Mukunda Stiles from the International Association of Yoga Therapists, but includes my own modifications. Prevention is always easier than cure, so I do recommend that you include at least some of these movements in the morning, working at your desk or at the end of your day. This slow conscious movement with slow breathing may help release muscle tension and stress through interoception and mental focus. (Watch the video on joint release for detailed instructions[*].)

Frozen shoulder

Frozen shoulder (also called adhesive capsulitis) is a common disorder that causes pain, stiffness and loss of normal range of motion in the shoulder. It mainly affects people aged 40–60 – and mostly women, possibly due to the decline in oestrogen causing inflammation, dehydration and loss of collagen.

When the shoulder becomes immobilized in this way, the connective tissue surrounding the glenohumeral joint – the joint capsule – thickens and contracts, losing its normal capacity to stretch. Pain also causes us to protectively tense our muscles so the humerus has less space to move in, and if we don't move the joint, it produces less lubricating synovial fluid.

If you think you have a frozen shoulder, consult your doctor before starting an exercise programme. They may recommend anti-inflammatory medication, ice packs to reduce inflammation around the

---

[*] https://www.youtube.com/playlist?list=PLJ-mltZchfBB9d6nOWWnOCaYHP4aQDOWC

joint, a corticosteroid injection and physiotherapy. Once the inflammation has reduced, practising shoulder stretches on a daily basis can help bring your mobility back. Please do not push yourself if you experience any pain.

Lower back pain

Back pain is now recognized as related to menopause for large numbers of women, especially those aged 45–60.[11]

Although the decline in oestrogen in perimenopause is an obvious cause, lower back pain is complex and can include everything from a sedentary lifestyle, posture and the way we sit, insomnia and our sleep position as well as depression and mental stress. What is now recognized by medical practitioners is that our emotions can contribute to lower back pain. Interestingly, there is a link between progesterone and our sensation of pain. Lower levels of progesterone may make us more sensitive to the sensation of pain, and our nervous system holds memory, so the pain you are experiencing today may be a primitive memory of a previous pain. The takeaway message from this is that this lower back pain is a loud message in our perimenopause that we need to treat our body with kindness and self-compassion. Pushing or forcing your way through the pain won't work.

Always consult your doctor if you experience these conditions. You may need an MRI to assess a spinal disc impingement or nerve damage.

5- to 15-minute practice

Knees to chest pose (apanasana), 10 times, alternating legs.

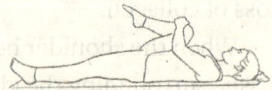

Windshield wiper twist pose (supta parivrtta sucirandhrasana), 8–10 times, slow, small movements left and right.

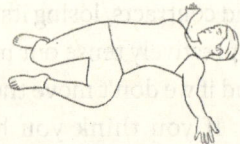

End with one of these restorative poses for 5–10 minutes.

Front lying savasana (adho mukha savasana), with folded blanket under hips.	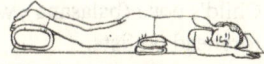
Supported child's pose (salamba balasana), with a bolster.	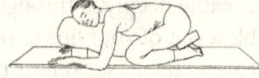

Sacroiliac joint pain

The sciatic nerve runs from your lower back through your buttocks, down the outside of your legs to your feet. If this nerve is irritated or compressed (trapped) it can cause pain all the way down to your leg, or 'pins and needles' tingling or numbness. If your symptoms include loss of bowel or bladder control and numbness that makes it difficult to stand or walk, you must seek urgent medical support. You may need an MRI to assess whether you have a spinal disc impingement or nerve damage.[12]

General advice to avoid sciatica includes:

- Stay hydrated.
- Sit evenly – avoid crossing your legs.
- Move more during your day, taking exercise snacks.
- Anti-inflammatory medication and HRT may help.
- Magnesium in the form of foods, creams and supplements may help relax your muscles.
- Sleep with a pillow or specialist hip support cushion between your legs to maintain joint stability.

Gentle massage and somatic movement is effective treatment for SI joint pain, according to a systematic review in the *Journal of Physical Therapy Science*.[13]

Here are some recommended yoga therapy movements that can help relieve discomfort, stretch the contracted muscles and reduce mental stress. The primary aim of these exercises is to alleviate the pain by gently stretching the area of muscle contraction and using your breathing to calm your nervous system to help your body relax.

Please note: Do not practise these if you have a disc impingement. You must see a physiotherapist and seek medical treatment.

5-minute practice

Child's pose (balasana), with knees together and forehead on fists.

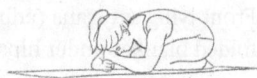

Breathe deeply in through your nose and gently blow out of your lips to relax your body and find ease in the pose. Repeat this style of breathing 10 times or more until you feel relaxed.

Caution: If you feel sharp nerve pain, stop the practice immediately.

Modifications: Place a folded blanket at your hip crease to create space between your thighs and chest in child's pose (balasana). Alternatively, if you want more support, place a pillow in the same place, or rest your chest on a bolster.

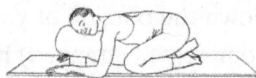

15-minute practice

Child's pose (balasana), with knees together and forehead on fists.

Pigeon pose (eka pada rajakapotasana). Start on the side with the sciatica pain first.

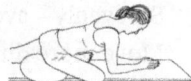

Side lying relaxation pose (modified savasana), with a pillow between your thighs.

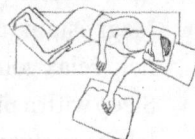

5- to 15-minute practice for sciatica due to a tight psoas muscle

Legs raised on pillows or bolster for Stonehenge relaxation pose (modified savasana) or on a chair (modified viparita karani). Lie on your back with a blanket underneath you for comfort. Place two or more pillows under the back of your knees and calf muscles so your legs are raised. This will relax your lower back muscles. Alternatively, rest your legs on a bolster raised on two blocks (Stonehenge relaxation pose), or rest your legs on a chair.

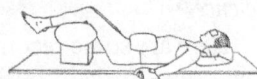

Please note: Always seek professional advice.

Sciatica due to the piriformis muscle

Your piriformis muscle is next to the sciatic nerve in your buttock, so the nerve may become squeezed in between the muscle, causing extreme pain.[14] These exercises are to stretch your buttocks to release the piriformis muscle and ease pressure off the sciatica nerve.

Supine thread the needle pose (urdhva mukha pasasana). Lie on your back with your legs bent and feet on the floor. Starting with the side that is not in pain, place your ankle on the other thigh, just below your knee, reach your arms through the gap between your legs, and gently hug towards your chest. Be gentle and stop if you experience any sharp nerve pain. Repeat 3 times and hold for 5–10 breaths, slowly in through your nose and exhale out of your mouth (ocean breath (ujjayi pranayama)). Then place both feet on the mat and notice if you feel any difference.

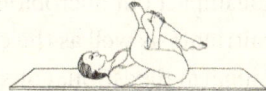

Piriformis diagonal stretch. Hug your knee to your chest and move your knee diagonally across your body, engaging your core muscles. This is not a spinal twist; the aim is to stretch the side of your buttocks. Hold for 5–10 slow breaths. Repeat on the other leg.

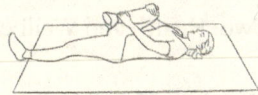

These poses may help you to rest and relax, which is essential if you have been in extreme pain and experiencing mental stress and loss of sleep. When the pain has gone, start building up strength in your core, gluteal muscles and pelvic floor, which create a stabilizing girdle around your lower back and pelvis.

Bloating and digestion

There are oestrogen receptors in your gut, and we now know more about the impact our microbiome has on our digestion, energy and absorption of nutrients as well as the enteric (gut) brain impact on our mental health. Sluggish digestion, constipation and bloating can also be accompanied by mental lethargy and low mood.

The bloating you may experience in perimenopause may feel similar to the water retention you felt in your monthly menstrual cycle, but lasting for longer than a few days. Food intolerances may arise, especially if inflammation in your digestive tract caused by low oestrogen is making it painful for you to digest certain foods. If you already have irritable bowel syndrome (IBS), then you may find this worsens. Generally speaking, an anti-inflammatory diet may be beneficial for you at this stage. (See Part Two: Health and Wellbeing, in particular the advice on nutrition.)

Caution: Bloating and abdominal pain may be a sign of a serious health condition such as a thickening of the womb lining, endometriosis, fibroids or cancer. Please always consult your doctor to rule out these risks before embarking on this yoga practice.

Bloating from gaseous wind

Gentle somatic movement and relaxing your nervous system with slow abdominal breathing will send a message to your digestive system that you are not in danger, so it can switch to a rest and digest mode. One simple way to release gas is to take a 10-minute walk, which may help balance blood sugar levels and move things along.

However, remember that chronic stress over time and the dehydration caused by low oestrogen may have caused a build-up and blockage of waste. This can cause excess gas that becomes trapped, and may be the cause of both bloating and constipation.

In this sequence, I have included breathing to relax your nervous system, gentle rhythmical twists and pressure on the ascending and descending colon to help shift waste and gas, and restorative poses that relax your whole abdomen and lower back psoas muscle group (the fight or flight muscles). The aim is to gently reassure your body and enteric brain that everything is okay, that it is safe to let go (of whatever waste needs to be released). This is a kind and compassionate way to bring your body out of muscle spasm of holding.

Caution: If you experience acid reflux or nausea lying down on your back, please stop the exercises and sit upright. Instead, practise supported relaxation pose (salamba savasana) with a raised bolster elevating your torso so your head is higher than your heart. Practise abdominal breathing (adham pranayama) until you feel better.

You may need to consult a doctor and nutritionist to look at your diet first, adding some soluble fibre to help assist your bowel movements. Return to this practice another day and make it a regular part of your daily practice, not just when you feel blocked. Over time, your digestive system will learn to relax on cue.

The poses in this section are inspired by my training with Charlotte Watts who is an expert in yoga therapy for digestive health, but also include my own modifications.[*]

5-minute practice

Abdominal breathing (adham pranayama) with ocean breath, for 20–30 breaths.	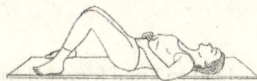

Box breathing (4-2-4-2). Repeat for 10 rounds.

15-minute practice
These poses are designed to help you release trapped digestive gas, so don't be surprised if you pass wind.

---

[*]   www.charlottewattshealth.com

Knees to chest pose (apanasana), aka wind-relieving pose, for 10 rounds. Hug both knees to your chest.

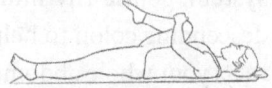

Windshield wiper twist pose (supta parivrtta sucirandhrasana) 10 times. Slow, small movements, side to side, with slow breathing.

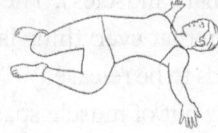

Child's pose-cat-cow (balasana-marjaryasana-bitilasana) flow, for 10 rounds.

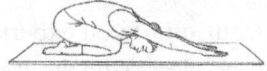

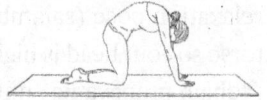

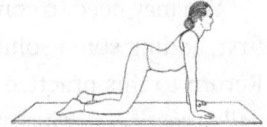

Child's pose (balasana), with ribs resting on the thighs, for 10 breaths.

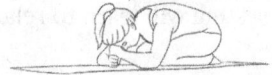

Sphinx pose (salamba bhujangasana), with abdomen supported by folded blanket, for 5 breaths.

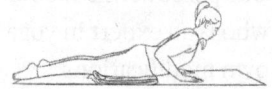

Low squat (malasana) for 5 breaths. Modify with heels supported by a blanket or a block.

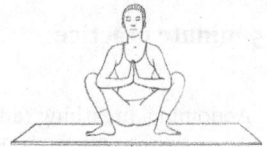

Head to knee forward fold (janusirsasana) or modify the pose.

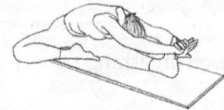

Watch these videos on digestive issues.*

_____

* https://www.youtube.com/playlist?list=PLJ-mltZchfBB9d6nOWWnOCaYHP4aQDOWC

30-minute practice

Finish with one of these restorative poses for 10–15 minutes.

Restorative legs raised on a chair or Stonehenge relaxation pose (modified savasana). If lying on your back is not comfortable (causes nausea), try alternative side lying relaxation pose (modified savasana) and supported twists, which help to relax your abdomen and stimulate peristalsis digestion.

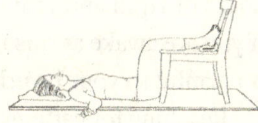

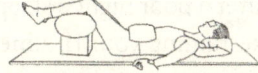

Restorative side lying poses and twists.

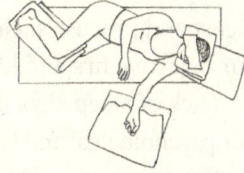

Journaling: Notice any movement of food or gas in your digestive tract. Has relaxing your abdomen with these poses helped to stimulate peristalsis or release wind? Do you feel less bloated or more alert, hungry even? Write down what poses worked best for you and add them to 'MY toolkit'. Keep a record of what you have consumed and whether this affects your bloating or constipation. We may become more sensitive to foods and drinks, for example wheat, sugar and alcohol.

Watch this video for a restorative lying twist[*]

MY CLASS FOR INSOMNIA AND SLEEP ISSUES

Sleep is essential to the human body and brain, and crucial for the healthy functioning of our bodily organs and tissues. Lack of sleep can cause higher cortisol (stress hormone) levels, and prevent effective digestion and elimination of food. Sleep deprivation prevents the brain from processing thoughts and experiences accumulated during the day, and can cause fatigue, inability to mentally focus or function at work, dizziness, loss of balance, headaches, low libido, irritability, low mood and

---

[*]   https://www.youtube.com/playlist?list=PLJ-mltZchfBB9d6nOWWnOCaYHP4aQDOWC

depression. Put simply, sleep resets and refreshes the body and brain. Without it, we cannot function.

Studies have shown that our body recharges and repairs between the hours of 11pm and 1am, which is when the gallbladder dumps its toxins. If you are awake at this time, these toxins are retained in the liver, which is harmful to your health.[15]

Reaching for caffeine, sugar and carbohydrates are common impulses after a poor night's sleep, which can, in turn, lead to a cycle of insomnia. Retraining your tiredness impulses is especially important during the menopause, because our metabolism slows down and we are less able to digest and process sugars and stimulants. In TCM and Ayurvedic terms, our digestive fire and kidneys become weaker.

Lack of sleep also affects our ability to dream, which is essential for our psychological and spiritual wellbeing. Remember: your body and brain are being transformed by the change in hormones at a cellular level during the menopause. Perimenopausal women need to sleep more – so why not give ourselves a pause in menopause? Radical rest is an act of self-care.

Here are some positive affirmations before bedtime:

> I am calm, I am safe, I am cared for.
> Everything is going to be okay.

'MY class for insomnia and sleep issues' is designed to prepare your body for a good night's sleep by using pandiculation, which is when we stretch our body and yawn at the same time. These are believed to tone or reset our vagal nerve, which helps us switch from the stress response (sympathetic nervous system) to rest and digest (parasympathetic nervous system).

'Jawning', a natural stress release

I start many of my classes for insomnia, fatigue and mood swings with yawning. Why? Because yawning is the body's own automatic stress-releasing mechanism before going to sleep. Notice how we usually stretch out our arms and legs before we yawn, and we open our jaw super-wide before we exhale with a yawn. This simple movement stretches the muscles in our body that hold stress-releasing lactic acid so our muscles can relax. The masticator muscles around the jaw are very strong in order to chew food, but in our perimenopause, we may notice our jaw feels tighter and we may wake up with a headache. Dentists recommend tooth guards, also known as mouthguards, during menopause to protect your teeth from damage caused by grinding or clenching when you sleep, a condition known as bruxism, which can be exacerbated by hormonal changes and stress. Yawning also stretches and tones the vagal nerve, which helps us switch from a stress response to rest and digest.

In summary, yawning is a simple stress-releasing mechanism that you can use to prepare you for sleep by releasing physical tension. Here is a practice that I call 'Jawning' because it starts with a gentle massage to relax tense jaw muscles and stimulate your yawn. In some cultures yawning in public may be viewed as rude, so you may want to practise this one at home!

If you are struggling with daytime fatigue, practise one of the restorative poses for 15–20 minutes in the afternoon.

5-minute practice

Ocean breath (ujjayi pranayama), sitting on your bed, for 5–10 breaths.

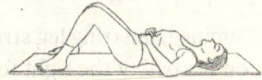

Circle your lower jaw clockwise a few times, then anticlockwise a few times.

Stretch your whole body and invite in a big jaw yawn, a 'jawn'.

Face massage. Use your fingertips to gently massage your temples, upper and lower jaw, chin, around your mouth and the bridge of your nose. Stretch the skin across your eyebrows and circle around your eyes softly. Stroke across your forehead, over your head, back of your head, back of your neck, front of your neck as you lift your chin, and cover your eyes with the palms of your hands.

Seated side stretches. Raise the right arm up and to the side, and then the left arm up and to the side.

Neck stretches. Lower the left ear towards the shoulder and then the right ear towards the shoulder.

15-minute practice

Constructive rest pose (savasana) and abdominal breathing (adham pranayama) with ocean breath, lying on your back on your bed, 8–10 times.

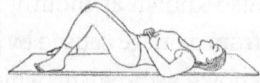

Full body stretch and yawn. If you don't feel a yawn, try tensing all your muscles for a few breaths, then releasing and relaxing.

Hug your knees to your chest.

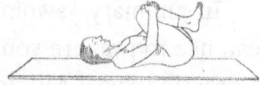

Knee circles, 10 times to stretch the inner thighs.

Half happy baby pose (modified ananda balasana), with right knee bent. Lie on your back and bend your right knee towards your chest. Reach your right arm inside of your leg and use your hand to hold the outside of your foot. If that is not accessible, loop a yoga strap over the ball of your foot. Draw your knee towards your right armpit and the sole of your foot facing the ceiling. This is a hip-opening stretch. Stay for a few breaths.

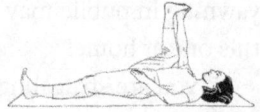

Supine hamstring leg stretch with a strap or belt on the ball of the right foot. Point and flex your foot a few times to stretch your hamstring, calf and Achilles tendon.

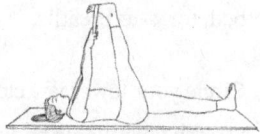

Hand to toe wide leg stretch to the right side using a strap and bolster for support. Stay for 5 breaths. This inner thigh stretch may trigger a 'jawn'.

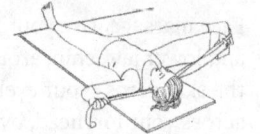

Half happy baby pose (modified ananda balasana), with other knee bent.

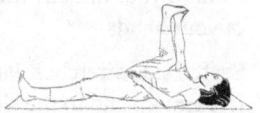

Supine hamstring leg stretch with other leg and a strap.

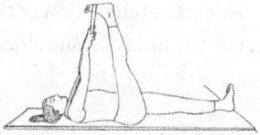

Hand to toe wide leg stretch to the other side, using a strap and bolster for support.

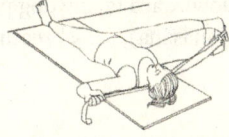

Bridge pose (setu bandha sarvangasana) flow. Feet hip distance apart. Exhale, roll up your spine towards your shoulder blades, inhale in bridge pose, exhale, roll down your spine. Repeat 5 times.

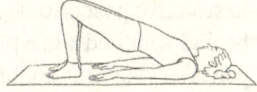

Windshield wiper twist pose (supta parivrtta sucirandhrasana), repeat 4 times on each side.

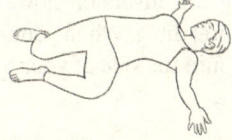

Constructive rest pose (savasana) with slow abdominal breathing (adham pranayama). Continue until you feel yourself drifting off to sleep.

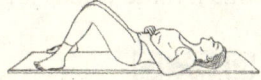

30-minute practice

If you are still feeling awake, add on this short sequence, ending with restorative pose (savasana).

Cat-cow-child's pose (marjaryasana-bitilasana-balasana) flow, 10 times.

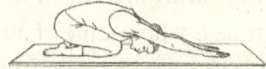

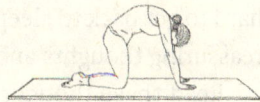

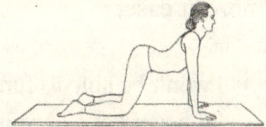

Sphinx pose (bhujangasana), for 5 breaths.

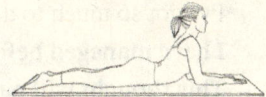

Extended child's pose (utthita balasana).

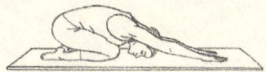

Downward facing dog pose (adho mukha svanasana), for 5 breaths.

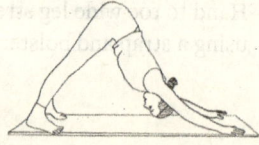

Restorative pose with legs raised up the wall behind your bed and a pillow underneath your pelvis so your hips are higher than your heart. Or stack some pillows underneath your knees. This gentle inversion slows down your heart rate and breathing. When you feel sleepy, simply roll over onto the side of your body and fall asleep.

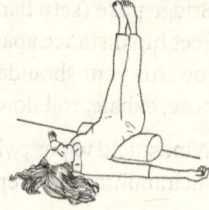

Watch these videos for sleep and insomnia.*

Cognitive behavioural therapy for insomnia

If you wake up regularly at night due to sweats, terror dreams or needing the bathroom, it can lead to anxiety and fatigue the next day. The night-time is when some of our darkest thoughts arise, only to seem trivial when we wake the next day. But if you are losing sleep every night and finding it hard to get back to sleep, you can try changing your catastrophizing into reassuring thoughts and remind yourself that you *can* cope.[16]

Read these thoughts below. Which set of thoughts makes you feel more at ease?

I won't be able to function tomorrow.

I'll never get a decent night's sleep again.

I've got so much to do tomorrow!

I have managed before so I know I can cope.

This thought will pass. Tomorrow, I can prioritize what is essential.

---

* https://www.youtube.com/playlist?list=PLJ-mltZchfBB9d6nOWWnOCaYHP4aQDOWC

MY CLASSES FOR FATIGUE
MY morning class for fatigue

If you have slept poorly, the next morning you may need an instant pick-me-up practice, so try one of these energizing breathing techniques. Choose one that works best for you and put it in your toolkit. (See 'Yoga basics: Breathwork'.)

5-minute practice

Lotus flower breath (padma pranayama). Sit on a chair with the soles of your feet on the floor. Rest your hands on your thighs and turn the palms of your hands up. Inhale through your nose as you open your hands wide, exhale through your nose as you gently close your hands. Repeat 3 rounds of 10 breaths.

You may notice that your nostrils flare open and close as you move your hands and your lungs expand more.

This gentle breathing technique encourages deeper breathing, which can be energizing. I like to visualize my palms moving like the petals of a lotus flower opening in the morning and closing at night.

Slow, gentle bellows breath (modified slow kapalabhati breathing), 3 rounds of 10 breaths.

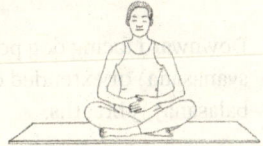

Breath of joy, 10 rounds.

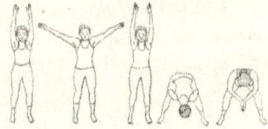

Alpha pose (urdhva hastasana) is a posture that increases your heart rate and deepens your breathing, which may feel energising, lift your mood and boost self confidence.

Instructions: stand with your legs wider than hip distance apart and your legs straight. Raise your arms up and your gaze upward for 5-10 breaths. Imagine that you are drawing energy from the sky down into your body. Slowly lower your arms and head, and notice if you feel more energised and positive.

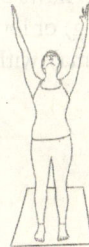

Remember to practise these gently and slowly, and pause in between each round to avoid dizziness.

15-minute practice

Standing side stretches, 4 times.

Half sun salutations (ardha surya namaskar), 5 times.

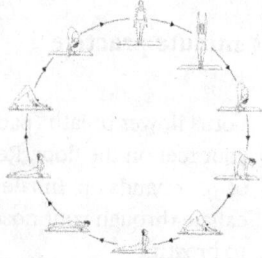

Meno-warrior chair pose squats (modified utkatasana), 10 times.

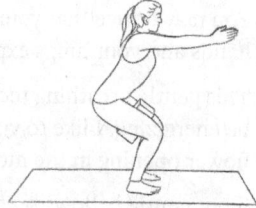

Downward facing dog pose (adho mukha svanasana) or extended child's pose (utthita balasana), 5 breaths.

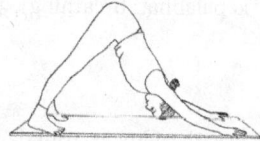

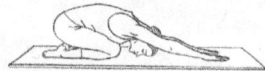

Seated bellows breath (slow kapalabhati breathing) or lotus flower breath (padma pranayama), with visualization, 3 rounds of 10 breaths.

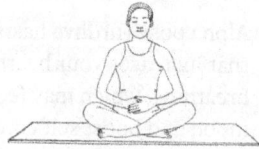

30-minute practice

Finish the 5- and 15-minute practice with this restorative pose.

Restorative mountain brook pose, 10 minutes.

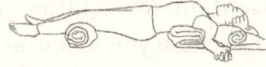

Watch the video on brain fog.[*]

MY afternoon class for fatigue

Instead of a food or exercise snack, nourish yourself with a sleep snack.

If you feel an energy slump mid-morning or afternoon, instead of tanking up with caffeine and sugar, which may increase your cortisol levels, give yourself instead a meno-*pause*, a 15-minute break to recharge your batteries. Rest really is best. Lisa Sanfilippo, author of *Sleep Recovery: The Five Step Yoga Solution to Restore Your Rest*, describes this as 'putting energy back on the grid'.[17]

Avoid going back to bed because this may confuse your body's natural circadian sleep rhythm and you need your mind to associate your bedroom with nighttime. Instead, practise one of the restorative yoga poses in my book. (See 'Restorative yoga poses'.)

Restorative legs raised on a chair.

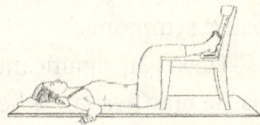

I recommend restorative legs raised up the chair, not a wall, but it is your choice. Cover your mat with a soft blanket and you can squish this around your neck and ears, and even cover your eyes and head if that feels cosy and comforting. Set a timer for 15 minutes and rest.

Tip: You can swap out the chair for a sofa, a coffee table or cushions. Support the back of your pelvis with a blanket or pillow so that your

---

[*]   https://www.youtube.com/playlist?list=PLJ-mltZchfBB9d6nOWWnOCaYHP4aQDOWC

hips are slightly higher than your heart; this slows down your heart and breathing rate, which tells your brain it is time to relax.

Caution: Avoid lifting your hips up onto a bolster – this is too high and may cause you to feel as if your blood is rushing to your head.

Avoid straightening your legs up a wall; in menopause you may experience vasomotor symptoms affecting your blood circulation, which can cause numbness or 'pins and needles' tingling in your feet and legs. This is not restful.

MY CLASS FOR HEALTHY WEIGHT

I am writing this section with some caution. My aim is not to body shame. Unrealistic body image is a misogynistic oppressive stick with which women have been beaten for centuries, so it has to stop here! Menopause is an opportunity for us to invite self-love and compassion by loving the bodies we are in; loving means nourishing in healthy ways that make us feel good. When we feel good, we look healthy and happy. So let's please start loving ourselves more.

Not everyone automatically gains weight at menopause, and HRT may cause you to gain or lose weight. Some adipose (fatty) tissue is actually good because it can be converted by your body into a low-grade version of oestrogen (oestrone), which may help ease some of your perimenopause symptoms.

However, significant weight gain around your midriff in postmenopause may become a health risk and indicator of future cardiovascular disease, breast cancer and type-2 diabetes. So we do need to manage our weight wisely, alongside strengthening our muscles, bones and brain.

Please note: If the information I have shared here triggers anxiety or negative health thoughts, please seek the support of a professional counsellor, or consult your doctor.

Why weight gain?

One of the reasons for weight gain is believed to be that our metabolism slows down as part of the ageing process, and our digestion becomes more sluggish, meaning it takes longer to digest and process the foods and drinks we consume. However, low oestrogen also plays a role in this change in weight distribution.

Muscle atrophy (sarcopenia) can change the appearance of your body, and adipose tissues burn fewer calories than muscle, so you may notice changes to your body shape even if your premenopause calorie intake hasn't changed. We need to add strength training to our weekly exercise so that we maintain or even build muscle to counter sarcopenia. Feeling strong can help us to feel more self-confident and may boost your daily energy.

However, the key is not to overdo it in menopause. Why? Because pushing our body too hard can cause fatigue and stress – and injury. Stress releases cortisol, which diverts energy away from the digestive organs because eating a big meal isn't seen as the priority in the primitive fight or flight mode. That is fine in the short run, but chronic long-term stress can keep your cortisol levels so high that you become less resistant to insulin, which makes you less able to lower your blood sugar levels after eating food. This, in turn, can cause more weight gain.

Insomnia and sleep issues (waking to go to the toilet/bathroom, night sweats and night terrors) may also increase weight gain (see 'MY class for insomnia and sleep issues'), and feeling fatigued the next day may lead us to make unhealthy food and drink choices (caffeine, sugar and processed carbs) to boost our energy, stimulating our stress response.

Learn gentle ways to reduce stress and include regular exercise 'snacks' to help you to reduce weight gain, lower your blood sugar levels and improve your sleep. Once you have your sleep and stress at healthier levels, you will have the energy to start strength training (see 'MY class for strength').

Research shows that women's bodies respond better to shorter bursts of exercise rather than longer workouts or running long distances.[18] The key is to conserve and use your energy wisely – don't deplete yourself.

Exercise for weight loss

Fitness coach Lavina Mehta MBE is an advocate of 'exercise snacking' – short bursts of activity throughout your day. I support Mehta's approach because we can all include a 5- minute exercise 'snack' or break in our day with a few squats, chair pose, lunges or lifting weights, and her 'exercise snacking' method is backed by research.

Research suggests that exercise snacking can improve fitness and reduce the risk of cancer and cardiovascular disease. Exercise snacking is defined as short bursts of physical activity throughout the day. Benefits include:

- Reduced risk of cancer and cardiovascular disease: A 2023 study in the *Journal of Sports Medicine* found that short bursts of activity were linked to a reduced risk of dying from cancer and cardiovascular disease.[19]
- Improved muscle strength: A study published in *Sports Medicine and Health Science* found that exercise snacks improved leg muscle strength and size in older adults.[20]
- Improved cardiovascular health: A review article published online by Stanford Lifestyle Medicine found that exercise snacks improved cardiorespiratory fitness.[21]

Mehta also includes yoga in her programme to help release myokines when we stretch – a feel-good hormone reward – which helps make movement motivating. Mehta does not recommend people eat less and work out more in the gym to manage weight in menopause because, she says, 'This will actually make the problem worse by overloading an already highly stressed body, with no time to apply any much-needed self-care, rest or recovery, which can lead to inflammation and further weight gain.'[22]

5- to 10-minute practice
Choose one, or all, of these poses for a quick exercise snack while you're waiting for the kettle to boil or to give yourself a computer screen break. I set a timer on my phone every hour to remind me to stand up and move.

Chair pose squats (utkatasana), with a brick between the thighs, 3 sets of 10. Add the meno-warrior arm movements for a fun sense of empowerment.

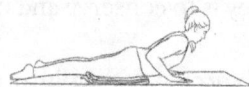

Mountain pose (tadasana), for 5 slow breaths. Use this pose to regulate your breathing and heart rate.

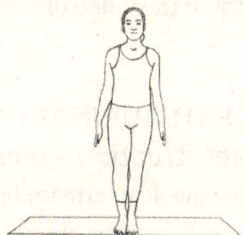

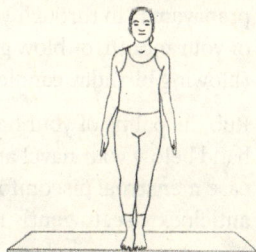

Step back lunges, 1 set of 10 lunges on alternating legs, followed by 10 lunges with the right leg and 10 lunges with the left leg. Swap the step back lunges for step forward lunges.

Always focus your weight into the heel of your front foot to boost balance and glute strength.

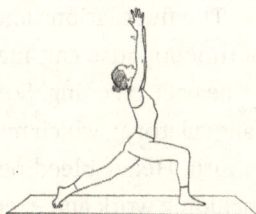

Mountain pose (tadasana), for 5 breaths.

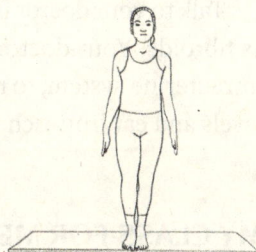

Goddess high squat pose (utkata konasana), pulsing for 10 breaths, then holding for 10 breaths.

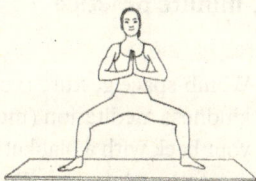

Mountain pose (tadasana), for 5 breaths. Use this pose to regulate your breathing and heart rate.

Tip: Add hand weights to these exercises – you'll be surprised how much weight you can hold, and it turbo-charges your glutes and thigh muscles.

Watch the video on weight gain.*

GENITOURINARY SYMPTOMS
Menstruation – menorrhagia

The medical term for heavy periods is menorrhagia, which can cause pain, muscle cramps, distress and fatigue.

The fluctuations and decline in oestrogen and progesterone during perimenopause can make your periods longer or shorter with lighter or heavier bleeding. Some months your ovaries may not release an egg (anovulatory), which means your menstrual bleed may be longer the next month. Heavy bleeding may negatively impact every area of your life, including work and exercise, and your social and sex life.

Talk to your doctor in case there is another gynaecological cause, such as fibroids. Your doctor may suggest you fit a Mirena coil, or a similar intrauterine system, to regulate your menstrual periods. Check your iron levels and eat iron-rich foods such as spinach.

MY CLASS FOR MENSTRUATION IN PERIMENOPAUSE
5-minute practice

Womb-space gesture (yoni mudra) and loving-kindness meditation (metta bhavana). Start on your back with a blanket underneath you for comfort and warmth. Begin ocean breath (ujjayi pranayama) in through your nose and sighing out of your mouth, or blow gently out of your lips (blowing birthday candle breath).

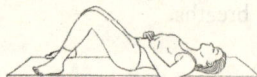

Rub the palms of your hands together to create warmth, then place one hand below your navel and one above. Allow the warmth of your hands to ease menstrual discomfort. Circle your hands clockwise, then circle them anticlockwise, to gently massage your abdomen.

Loving-kindness meditation (metta bhavana). Repeat for 5 minutes.

---

* https://www.youtube.com/playlist?list=PLJ-mltZchfBB9d6nOWWnOCaYHP4aQDOWC

Womb-space gesture (yoni mudra). Some people find this very powerful for creating a healing energy and intention.

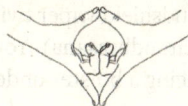

15-minute practice

Cat-cow-child's pose (marjaryasana-bitilasana-balasana) flow, with hip circles clockwise and anticlockwise, for 5 minutes.

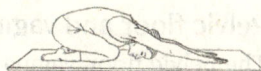

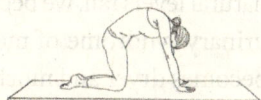

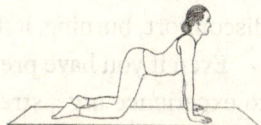

Supported child's pose (utthita balasana), with a bolster and blocks.

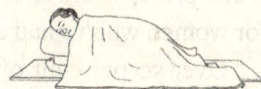

Optional: You may like to place a blanket to cover your whole back, or fold the blanket and wrap around your lower back, around your kidneys. This can feel warm and comforting to help ease menstrual pain.

Modification: If child's pose is painful for your knees, lie on your back and hug the bolster, either crossing your ankles over the bolster or resting the soles of your feet against a wall.

Additional restorative poses

For the days when you don't feel like putting any pressure on your abdomen, you can practise these restorative poses.

Restorative side lying twist (salamba supta matseyandrasana), with blankets and eye pillow (see 'Restorative yoga poses'). Stay for 5–10 minutes on the left and then the right side.

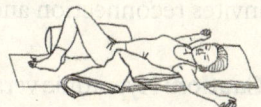

Windshield wiper twist pose (supta parivrtta sucirandhrasana). You can make it restorative by placing a bolster under your legs.

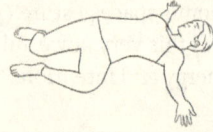

MY CLASS FOR PELVIC FLOOR STRENGTH
Pelvic floor and vaginal atrophy

The pelvic floor, vagina and vulva are dependent on oestrogen. As our natural levels fall, we become more prone to a condition known as 'genito-urinary syndrome of menopause', or GSM for short. The vaginal lining becomes dryer and much more delicate. This can lead to discomfort during sex, bleeding after sex, recurrent urine infections, thrush, generalized discomfort, burning, itching and bladder weakness.

Even if you have previously had a healthy pelvic floor, you may start to experience urge, stress or faecal incontinence. Uterine, bladder and rectal prolapse are another reality, and there are special considerations for women who've had a hysterectomy.

Over 50 per cent of menopausal women experience some kind of incontinence at menopause. Incontinence can be a barrier to exercise at a time when moving our body is key to staying healthy. Changes to the pelvic floor muscles can be destabilizing and impact your self-esteem.

> *When the pelvis no longer feels like a familiar or safe place to rest your attention, when you are worried about whether or not you will make it to the toilet on time, if you are going to leak when you sneeze, or whether you will enjoy giving and receiving pleasure during love making, you can feel very vulnerable.*
>
> (JESSICA ADAMS, WOMEN'S HEALTH PRACTITIONER)

Trauma may also be held in the pelvis, and can come to the surface at menopause. This is why it's so important to nurture your connection to this area of your body, one that extends beyond pelvic floor exercises and invites reconnection and the potential for deep healing.[23]

Caution: Hypotonic versus hypertonic pelvic floor muscles. Not everyone develops weaker pelvic floor muscles (hypotonic) after menopause. Some people have tightly contracted pelvic floor muscles (hypertonic), which can also cause pain and problems with sexual intercourse and passing urine and faeces. If you have overactive pelvic floor muscles, please avoid the strengthening class in this book, and instead focus on relaxing the pelvis with gentle hip-opening yoga poses and abdominal breathing. (See 'MY class for hot flushes and night sweats', and 'Bloating and digestion'.)

You are recommended to seek medical diagnosis for pelvic floor conditions and you may need individualised professional support.

This practice is for women who have hypotonic weaker pelvic floor muscles due to menopause. The fascia of the pelvic floor declines by around 4 per cent every year after the age of 40, so strengthening the leg muscles and the 64 muscles that are connected to the pelvis is also essential for maintaining integrity as women age. However, healthy pelvic muscles need the 'tone' or elasticity to contract and tighten when needed, and also to relax to avoid a hypertonic pelvis.[24] Please use the lotus flower visualization during this practice. This breathing technique is demonstrated in the pelvic floor class video.

10-minute practice, for morning and evening

Start by lying on your back. Place a yoga brick or block in between your thighs; this engages your pelvic floor muscles more and protectively stabilizes your sacroiliac joint.

Pelvis circles, clockwise on your mat 10 times and anticlockwise 10 times. This starts to engage your abdominal muscles and massages your lower back.

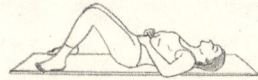

Pelvic tilts. Inhale as you tilt your tailbone down to the mat, which will create a small arch in your lower back. Exhale as you tilt your tailbone up, which will flatten your lower back towards the mat. Slowly rock up and down with your tailbone, moving with your breath.

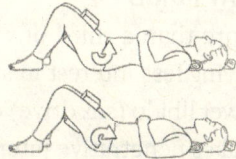

Lotus flower visualization. Visualize a lotus flower (or your favourite flower) at your perineum (between your anus and vulva). Every time you exhale, tilt your tailbone up and imagine closing the flower petals into a tight bud and draw it in and upwards. Every time you inhale, tilt your tailbone down and imagine the flower petals opening as you relax your pelvic floor.

Bridge pose (setu bandha sarvangasana) flow (slowly and sequentially). Exhale, tilt your tailbone up, close the flower bud and roll up your spine, just a few vertebrae. Keep your flower bud closed as you inhale in a low bridge pose and exhale as you slowly roll down your spine. When your pelvis touches the mat, inhale deeply, open your flower petals and relax your pelvic floor. Repeat 5–10 times, sequentially rising higher up your spine into a full bridge pose.

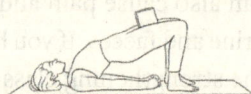

Constructive rest pose (savasana) with abdominal breathing and ocean breath, 5–10 times. Relax your pelvic floor muscles using abdominal breathing (adham pranayama) and ocean breath (ujjayi pranayama).

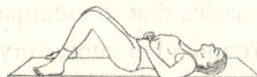

Remember: Healthy pelvic tone is the ability to relax and contract at will.

Windshield wiper twist pose (supta parivrtta sucirandhrasana). Gently lower your knees to the left and then the right in small, slow movements. This will also help relax your abdomen. Roll over on to one side of your body and come up to a seated position.

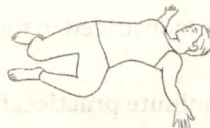

Watch the video on pelvic floor health.*

MY CLASS FOR LOW LIBIDO
Low libido

More than a third of women in perimenopause or menopause report having less interest in sex and trouble having an orgasm. Women report lower libido (sex drive) during perimenopause and vaginal dryness, which makes penetrative intercourse painful.[25]

The decline in oestrogen affects your vaginal biome, changing the PH level, causing vaginal dryness and thinning of vaginal tissues, which can make penetrative sex painful and trigger urinary tract infarctions. This also affects your ability to feel sexually aroused.

Localized HRT oestrogen pessaries strengthen the skin and rebalance

---

* https://www.youtube.com/playlist?list=PLJ-mltZchfBB9d6nOWWnOCaYHP4aQDOWC

the PH levels. However, testosterone also helps maintain muscle tone and is prescribed by doctors for women (and men) for low libido. Hormone treatments may not be safe for women with a history of breast cancer, so always consult your doctor.

Cardiovascular movement increases blood circulation and lifts your mood. Lifting weights can boost your energy and body self-confidence. Use a dildo vibrator for self-stimulation to tone the muscles you need to orgasm. These are the same muscles that strengthen and support your pelvic floor.

This class is similar to 'My class for pelvic floor strength', but instead of flowing up and down your spine, you focus on contracting your perineum (flower) in and upwards while keeping your pelvis on the mat. The aim is to hold for longer while breathing in and out of your nose. There is an option to squeeze the brick or block between your thighs, if this helps you to feel your pelvic muscles.

This class also includes the lotus flower mudra (padma mudra) hand movements and breathing.

Remember: Being able to relax your pelvic floor muscles is as important as toning them.

5-minute practice

Start by lying down on your mat or bed in a constructive rest pose (savasana). Place your arms alongside your body, with your palms facing up. Inhale through your nose, open your hands and relax your pelvic floor muscles. Exhale though your nose, close your hands into gentle fists, and zip in and up from your anus to your urethra, as if trying to stop the flow of urine on the toilet.

Repeat for 3 rounds of 10 breaths. Then relax, breathe naturally and notice how you feel.

Progress by holding the squeezes for longer, but don't hold your breath!

20- to 30-minute practice

Finish your practice with this restorative pose using as many props as you need for maximum support and comfort. The aim is not to stretch or strain; you want your hips and groin area to relax.

Queen reclined supported cobbler pose (rani salamba supta baddha konasana). This pose gently opens the front of the pelvis to stretch the abdomen and supports the lumbar spine, so this can relieve muscle cramps caused by menstruation.

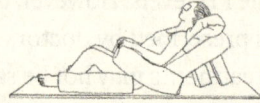

It is important to support the knees and legs as you open the hips, to prevent overstretching the groin.

Self-massage with oils (abhyanga)

The benefits of practising this ancient Ayurvedic self-massage therapy are that you are nourishing your skin with essential oils, stimulating your blood and lymph circulation while practising an act of self-care and love, and befriending your emotions about your changing body – and the sensation of smooth touch may stimulate your arousal. In essence it involves massaging yourself from head to toe using warmed-up essential oils.

Self-massage helps you to tune into your changing body. Loving your body can help you to feel more confident with your sexual partner. (See the section on self-massage in Part Two: Health and Wellbeing.)

MY CLASS FOR BLADDER WEAKNESS
Urinary tract infections, bladder weakness and urge incontinence

Urinary tract infections (UTIs) are caused by bacteria and may become more frequent in postmenopause, along with bladder weakness and urge incontinence.

Stress affects your vagina and bladder biome, elasticity and function. High levels of stress can reduce your body's immune system, which can, in turn, heighten your risk of developing an infection. According to the National Association for Continence, people with an overactive bladder need the bathroom more often when they are feeling stressed.[26] If this occurs at night, interrupted sleep can also weaken your immune system in a vicious circle.

There are several types of urinary incontinence. Stress incontinence is when urine leaks out at times when your bladder is under pressure; for example, when you cough or laugh. Urge (urgency) incontinence is when you feel a sudden urge to pee and urine leaks out. This is partly due to weaker pelvic floor muscles and bladder atrophy caused by declining oestrogen, progesterone and testosterone. Instead of fully emptying our bladder when we go to the toilet, our weak muscles do not squeeze out all of the liquid held in pockets of these slack muscles.

Practise 'MY class for pelvic floor strength' and 'MY class for low libido'. The perineum muscles you engage to urinate are the same.

Menopause Yoga for long-term health

Do you want to survive postmenopause or thrive in your Second Spring?

Women live on average until their mid-80s – that's approximately 30 years after menopause, which is a third of your life! Do you want to thrive or just survive in those 30 years?

From the age of 50+, our risk of developing serious health conditions increases as we age. The leading causes of death are dementia and Alzheimer's disease, coronary heart disease, diabetes and breast cancer. However, other conditions impact our quality of life: one in two women in postmenopause are at risk of developing osteoporosis (brittle bones) and sarcopenia (muscle atrophy), which affects our mobility and independence, and may exacerbate depression, lethargy (extreme fatigue) and loss of joy (anhedonia), which may lead to low self-confidence and social withdrawal. So, staying healthy, active and socially connected is key to enjoying our postmenopause years.

In this section we look at long-term health, and I offer some yoga and exercise practices for:

- Cancer
- Bone health*
- Balance and proprioception
- Muscle strength
- Heart health.

---

* Yoga is beneficial to bone density as part of a holistic package that includes strength training and nutrition.

Caution: Although these are self-practice classes, I encourage you to first seek one-to-one support from a physiotherapist and yoga teacher who specializes in your condition.

YOGA FOR CANCER

Yoga may help some people with cancer cope with managing their emotional wellbeing while waiting for treatment and aid mobility after treatment, including surgery. A systematic review of 18 research studies concluded that yoga can be beneficial in alleviating the fatigue-pain-sleep disturbance symptom cluster in breast cancer patients.[27]

Physical activity is recommended by cancer support organizations to both prevent and reduce future risk of breast cancer, because movement helps reduce the level of circulating hormones associated with breast cancer development. Gentle yoga stretches may also improve range of movement after surgery, building physical confidence as part of recovery.[28]

> Yoga has become an essential part of my life following a breast cancer diagnosis during menopause. Yoga was critical to my mental and physical wellbeing leading up to my mastectomy – the routines, the breathing and the poses were calming, strengthening and resilience building. Then following surgery, yoga was responsible for the return of full movement and recovery in my chest and shoulder. Since then, I have continued to use yoga for strength, flexibility and relaxation – now if I don't do yoga I feel weaker and less resilient. In addition, the side effects of post-cancer preventative medicine are similar to those in menopause, so yoga can help with dealing with these whilst building strength to counter bone density changes.
>
> Caroline wilkinson

Here is 'MY class for breast cancer recovery', and for a wider range of practices I recommend attending specialist Yoga for Cancer classes with a teacher such as Jenni Stone,* who provides personalized support, and there are also social benefits in meeting other people going through similar treatment.

---

* See www.jennitherapy.com

MY CLASS FOR BREAST CANCER RECOVERY

In the lead-up to and during your medical treatment, learning to regulate your nervous system may help reduce stress and anxious thoughts. 'MY class to reduce stress' and 'MY class for anxiety' will be beneficial, and the CBT exercises may also help. The best place to start is simply with your breath. (See 'Yoga basics: Breathwork'.)

If you have had breast surgery, you are advised to wait until the stitches and tissues have healed before starting the exercises. A simple massage of the affected tissues to improve blood circulation in this area will help the healing process and your emotional connection to this part of your body, which may be associated with pain.

The research shows that physical exercise and movement reduces cancer recurrence, but you may still feel fatigued, especially after chemotherapy or radiotherapy, so avoid overexerting or you could deplete your energy.[*] I have listed a couple of restorative poses, modified breathing and meditation techniques here, and the short 5- to 15-minute classes for muscle strength, bones and balance could help too. (See 'Restorative yoga poses', and 'MY class for strength'.)

Mind–body connection and alleviating anxiety

5-minute practice

Start seated or lying on your back in constructive rest pose (savasana) with abdominal breathing (adham pranayama) and ocean breath (ujjayi pranayama). Repeat 10 times, with a long, slow exhalation each time.

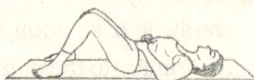

Positive affirmation: Repeat this 10 times, either speaking out loud, or in your mind if you are in a public place: 'I am safe. I am well cared for. I care for myself.' Or alternatively: 'I can get through this, one breath at a time.'

Journaling: Afterwards, if it feels safe for you, notice how you feel in your body – where do you feel it? Can you name that sensation? How is your breathing (fast and shallow or slower, deeper)? How active is your mind? Are your thoughts scattered or quieter? How do you feel emotionally? Can

---

[*] See www.breastcancer.org/treatment/complementary-therapy/types/yoga

you give this feeling a name? Use your journal to write down the words you have chosen to describe how you feel. Do this without judgement or expectation; every day or every hour may feel different. This is an important part of interoception – reconnecting mind and body. It is also a reminder that our feelings change constantly, so how we feel now will pass.

Caution: If you do not feel safe practising this interoception, please *stop*. Do whatever reduces your stress response (e.g., move your body, walk outside, take long, slower exhalations) and bring yourself back to a place of personal safety. You can return to this yoga practice another day, when you are ready.

15-minute practice

Restorative legs raised on a chair. If you are experiencing body heat from chemotherapy and your skin is sensitive, avoid placing a blanket over your body or the head cocoon, unless you feel cold.

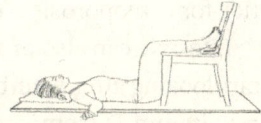

Tip: A weighted eye bag on your forehead can feel calming and grounding.

Yoga after chemotherapy

Chemotherapy creates heat in the body that may feel like a burning sensation or cause your skin to feel sensitive to touch. Unlike the hot flushes that come and go in menopause, this chemo heat and sensitivity may persist for weeks and months, so finding ways to feel ease is essential. As a yoga therapist, I suggest you practise cooling breathing (pranayama) and poses to release physical heat and calm your mind. Watch these videos on cooling hot flushes[*] and see 'Yoga basics: Breathwork'.

---

[*]   https://www.youtube.com/playlist?list=PLJ-mltZchfBB9d6nOWWnOCaYHP4aQDOWC

OSTEOPOROSIS

Osteoporosis is a condition where the bones lose strength, making you more likely to fracture a bone. Risk of developing osteoporosis increases as we age, but impacts women more than men.

Osteoporosis creates large honey-comb cavities in the bones that weaken the structure, making bones more fragile to fracture. Common areas affected are the hips, spine and wrists. Osteopenia is the less severe stage of weakened bones before reaching osteoporosis.

Osteoporosis in women may be due to the sharp decline in oestrogen for the first five years after the menopause. People who have a family history of osteoporosis, and women who have an early menopause or their ovaries removed as a result of a hysterectomy are at higher risk.

Oestrogen facilitates the growth of new bone material, so osteopenia may be reversed with HRT by replacing this hormone. The results of using HRT for osteoporosis are less clear.

Lifestyle can also protect bone density declining, and the earlier you start looking after your bones, the better. A diet rich in protein, calcium and vitamin D from sunlight (or supplements in winter) and phyto-estrogens (see the section 'Nutrition' in Part Two: Health and Wellbeing) may help prevent or stabilize osteoporosis.

> Your bones get bored – they are a living part of your body that need stimulating challenges and positive physical stress with progressive loading.
>
> Petra Coveney

Weight-bearing and muscle-strengthening exercises, such as lifting weights and jogging, apply positive stress on your bones, which respond by replacing old bone with new material. Bones get bored and respond well to stimulating challenges, so progressive loading exercise is seen to be the most effective approach. You can also use Pilates resistance bands that work by using small muscle and ligament movements in your joints to stimulate bone growth. This may release myokines, which make you feel good.

Strength training

Starting with your own body weight, you can gradually build up using a Pilates resistance band and then add handheld weights to your exercise routine as you start to feel stronger. (See 'MY class for strength'.)

YOGA FOR BONE HEALTH

Yoga alone cannot strengthen your bones, but it *can* help reduce stress and improve sleep, which both have an impact on bone density. Yoga can also help you develop core muscle tone and balance (proprioception) to prevent falls, leading to bone fractures, as well as an upright spinal posture to prevent osteoporotic kyphosis (a rounded back and shoulders).

Yoga stretches also bring other benefits. They create micro tears in your muscle tissue that stimulate your muscle cells to repair by growing new muscle fibres – thereby making you stronger! The release of skeletal muscle myokine[29] proteins may also have a positive endocrine effect.

Fitness trainer and health campaigner Lavina Mehta MBE says that stretching releases feel-good hormones, called endorphins, which help you feel positive and reduce pain.[30]

Yoga is also a good gateway or starting point for exercise, especially if you have been inactive or are recovering after an injury. When you've gained confidence in your mind–body coordination, you may feel ready to join group exercise classes, such as lifting weights and resistance training, which can boost bone density.

I use weights in my own daily routine, and include hand dumbbells for strength and balance classes with my private clients. This has complemented my yoga practice by strengthening my legs and gluteal muscles, and my abdominal 'core muscles' that improve balance postures such as tree pose (vrksasana).

So, although yoga may not increase bone density, it can build balance, core strength and stability, and the stretch element of many yoga poses may help muscles repair and strengthen after exercise, boost your mood and help you to feel relaxed. By reducing stress and improving sleep, you are helping to prevent future bone density loss.

I let go of the notion that osteoporosis happened to old-aged pensioners when I was diagnosed with osteopenia at 37 and osteoporosis at 45. I believed thinning bones occurred in old age but came to understand that it was in fact a disease of mid-life – a 'silent thief' that would steal my bone and leave me at risk of fracture.

Even if you don't have an osteoporosis diagnosis, do everything you can to support your bones and make stress reduction a priority.

I have adapted my yoga practice and nourish my bones with healthy foods, exercise and being in Nature. I visualize my bones shining brightly, sparkling and pulsing with light! When I meditate, I send them love, prana and healing energy.

Love your bones, nurture them, nourish them, and support them so they can support you too.

Sarah Thomas, yoga teacher for bone health[*]

Yoga modifications for osteoporosis

Watch the video on yoga modifications for osteoporosis.[**]

- Forward folds. Avoid rounding your back in standing or seated forward folds, head or shoulder stand and plough pose (halasana). Instead, bend your knees and hinge at your hips, keeping your spine straight. Head stand, shoulder stand and plough pose should be avoided.
- Sitting. Ensure your hips are higher than your knees, and avoid tucking your tailbone. You need to create space between your sit bones.
- Twisting. Use your abdominal muscles to rotate your spine. Avoid hooking your elbow over your knee to force yourself into the twist.
- Backbends. Practise spinal extensions to strengthen the muscles along your back that give you an upright posture.
- Balance poses are good to prevent falling. Strengthen your core abdominal muscles for stability.

SARAH THOMAS' AFFIRMATION FOR BONE HEALTH

My bones are filled with prana, my bones are filled with joy.
My bones are strong and flexible.
My bones are filled with vitality and healing energy flows freely through them.

---

[*] https://bewellbeingyou.co.uk/about-sarah-3
[**] https://www.youtube.com/playlist?list=PLJ-mltZchfBB9d6nOWWnOCaYHP4aQDOWC

MY CLASS FOR BALANCE

Here are some simple yoga poses that are designed to build your balance by improving your proprioception, and engaging your core abdominal muscles for pelvic stability. There are also poses to improve your posture to prevent the hyperkyphosis of extreme osteoporosis in the spine.

Feet are your foundation for posture, balance and a sense of stability. If we fracture a bone in later life, it may take longer to heal, and if you have osteoporosis, it can lead to long-term immobility, which affects our bones and leads to muscle atrophy. So, maintaining balance is essential for your long-term health and mobility, ultimately affecting your independence and sociability.

Include these simple balance poses in your daily life – when you are brushing your teeth or waiting for the kettle to boil, standing at a bus stop or in a supermarket queue.

5-minute practice

Warm-up: joint mobilizing sequence (pawunmuktasana).

Watch the video on joint release.* Stand on one leg and lift the other foot off the floor. Circle your foot clockwise a few times and then circle it anticlockwise. Point and flex your foot a few times. This warms up your ankle joints to prepare for balance. Place this foot on the mat and lift all your toes off the mat. Spread the toes wide. This will engage the arch of your foot. Starting with your little toe, slowly lower them all to the mat. Notice how this foot feels more connected to the ground now.

Repeat on the other foot.

Heel raises. Raise both your heels up as you inhale and down as you exhale to stretch and strengthen the three layers of arch muscles in your feet. Repeat 10 times.

Beginners: Sit in a chair and raise your heels.

Tip: Inhale, raise both arms as you inhale to lift your heels, and exhale as your lower your arms and heels.

---

* https://www.youtube.com/playlist?list=PLJ-mltZchfBB9d6nOWWnOCaYHP4aQDOWC

Mountain pose (tadasana) with tree roots visualization. (Watch my video on balance.) Stand with both feet on the floor. Spread your toes wide to open the soles of your feet to the floor. Root down into your feet to feel a connection with the Earth beneath you. Imagine you are a tree growing roots through the soles of your feet down into the soft earth beneath you. Strengthen your legs, lengthen your spine, lift the crown of your head towards the sky, take a deep breath in through your nose, and as you exhale, slide your shoulder blades softly down your back. Close your eyes (if you are not dizzy) and take 3–4 slow breaths.

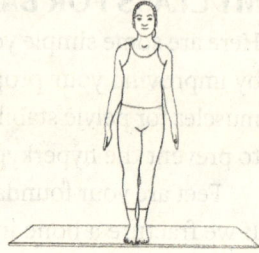

Balance challenge on one leg. Stand on one leg and raise the other knee. Bend the standing leg and pulse up and down 10 times. Repeat on the other leg. This builds balance, and engages your knee ligaments and muscles in the thighs and glutes. Strong legs means stability. Repeat 10 pulses on each leg.

Beginners: Place one hand lightly onto a chair or wall for balance.

Tip: Press the palms of your hands together; this helps you to balance.

Chair pose squats (modified utkatasana), with heel lifts and a brick or block in between the thighs. Repeat 5–10 times.

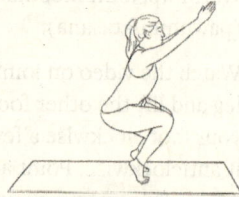

Mountain pose (tadasana). Start with the previous version of mountain pose, with eyes closed, if this feels safe and stable for you. Remember the tree roots from your feet that are grounding you and keeping you stable. Shift your weight slightly to the right side of your feet, then the left, and then shift forward towards your toes and back towards your heels. Circle your weight around the outside edges of your feet clockwise, and then anticlockwise. Find a place that feels balanced in the centre for you (we are all a bit wonky in leg length). Take 10 slow breaths before opening your eyes. This develops your proprioception (a sense of your body in the space around you), which is essential for balance.

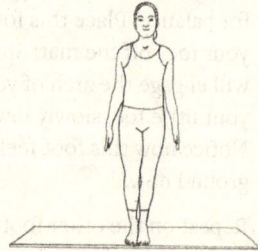

Beginners: You can practise these sitting on the edge of a chair or standing with the wall behind you for support.

Meno-warrior chair pose squats (modified utkatasana) to standing balance with heel lifts, 4–8 times. Sit into chair pose, squeezing a brick between your thighs, and lift your heels. Keep your heels lifted as you straighten your legs, balancing on the balls of your feet for 2–4 seconds, then lower your heels to stand upright.

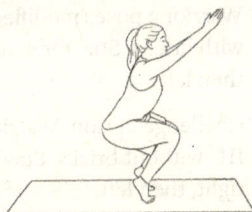

Beginners: Sit to stand using a chair. Sit on the edge of a chair and stand up 10 times without using your arms to lift you. This strengthens your legs and abdominal muscles.

Seated tree meditation and breathing. Sit on a chair with the soles of your feet touching the ground. Root down into your sit bones and lengthen your spine. Place your hands with palms down on your thighs. Close your eyes.

Tree meditation: Allow your abdomen to be relaxed so that you can breathe more deeply. As you breathe slowly, imagine you are inhaling through the soles of your feet (tree roots), travelling up your legs (tree trunk) to your belly, rib cage, chest and lungs (tree branches), and then all the way back down to the soles of your feet (tree roots). See if you can make your exhale longer than your inhale. For example, breathe in for the count of 1, 2, 3, 4 and exhale 1, 2, 3, 4, 5 or 6. If this makes you feel tense, go back to natural breathing at your own pace. Continue for 10 rounds of breath. Then notice how you feel. This tree breathing meditation can help you feel more grounded.

Tip: If your back becomes tired, place a bolster or firm pillow behind you for support.

30-minute practice

Warrior 3 pose (modified virabhadrasana III), with pulsing.

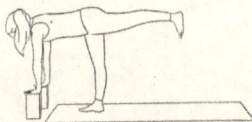

Mountain pose (tadasana), for 4 breaths.

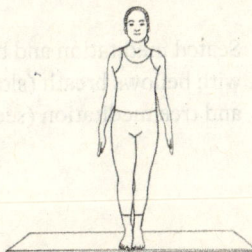

Warrior 3 pose (modified virabhadrasana III), with bricks. Stay for 5–10 breaths each leg, right then left.

Challenge option: Warrior 3 pose (virabhadrasana III) without bricks. Stay for 5–10 breaths each leg, right, then left.

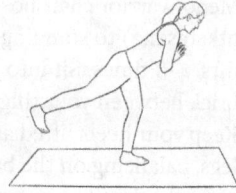

Tree pose (vrksasana). Stay on the left leg for 10 breaths, then stand in mountain pose (tadasana). Change legs to balance on the right leg for 10 breaths.

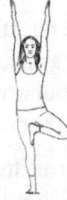

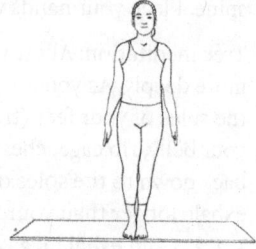

Standing pigeon pose (tada kapotasana). Stay for 4–5 breaths balancing on your left leg, then stand up and change to balance on your right leg for 4–5 breaths.

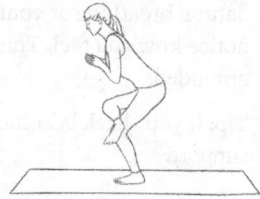

Mountain pose (tadasana), for 4 breaths. Circle your ankles and shake your legs if your muscles feel tight.

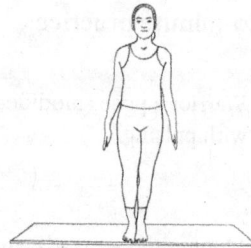

Seated meditation and breathing, for example with bellows breath (slow kapalabhati breathing) and tree meditation (see above).

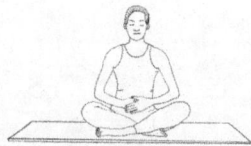

Watch the videos on balance.*

MY CLASS FOR STRENGTH

Yoga can help you maintain your muscle mass[31] by reducing stress, improving sleep and toning specific muscle groups with longer held hatha poses. We love feeling stronger, and can balance and hold yoga poses for longer, which also benefits our heart health and develops mental and emotional resilience.

> Yoga is a gateway, building confidence for you to attend other higher-intensity strength exercise classes. Technique is important for avoiding injury, so always seek guidance from a professional personal trainer and your doctor before embarking on a new exercise.

5-minute practice

Meno-warrior chair pose squats (modified utkatasana), 10 times.

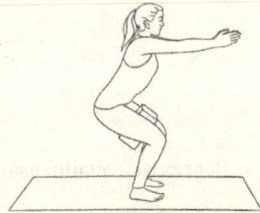

Chair pose squats (modified utkatasana), with pulsing, 10 times.

Mountain pose (tadasana), for 2–4 breaths.

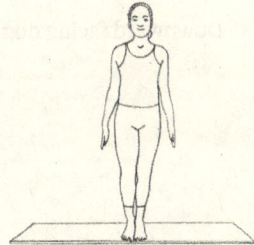

---

* https://www.youtube.com/playlist?list=PLJ-mltZchfBB9d6nOWWnOCaYHP4aQDOWC

Modified sun salutation (surya namaskar):

- Plank pose (phalankasana)

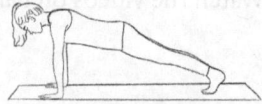

- Cobra pose (bujangasana)

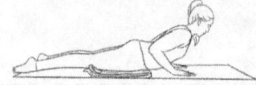

- Child's pose (balasana) or downward facing dog pose (adho mukha svanasana)

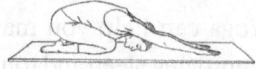

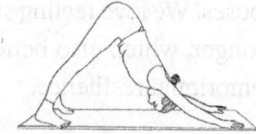

- Plank pose, hold for 10 breaths

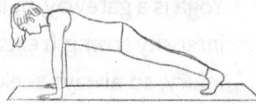

- Modified table top pose (bharmanasana), with micro press-ups or knee press-ups, 10 times

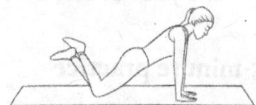

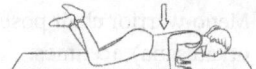

- Bear pose (bhallukasana), for 5–10 breaths

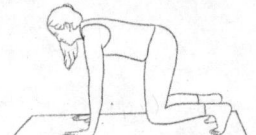

- Downward facing dog pose, for 5 breaths

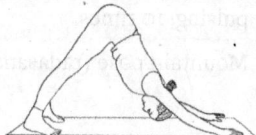

- Locust pose (salabhasana), for 5 breaths

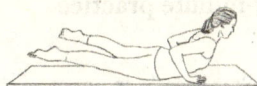

- Low cobra pose, lifting chest, arm and legs on exhale. Repeat 2–5 times

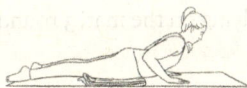

- Plank pose with shoulder taps, 4–10 times. Option: Table top pose with shoulder taps

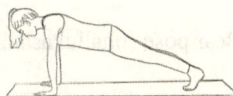

- Child's pose, for 5 breaths

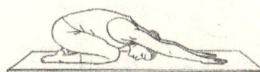

- Side plank twist variations: Supported side plank on right forearm and with left foot in front of the body; full side plank: thread the upper arm through the lower arm, 5 times each side. Swap to the other arm and leg

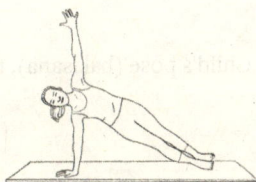

- Child's pose for 10 breaths, before sitting upright

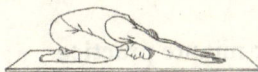

Additional poses: Swap out one of the chair poses for warrior 2 pose (virabhadrasana II) for 10 slow breaths (approx. 1 minute), each side.

Abdominal core stability

Your 'core' is the short-hand name for the deep abdominal muscles at the centre of your body that support your pelvis, back and spine. Think of the area from your lower ribs down to your pubic bone that mesh together and wrap around your mid to lower back. When they are toned and engaged it can feel like you are wearing a girdle that gives you upright posture. This is important for preventing lower back pain and the hyper-kyphosis rounding of your back that results from lifestyle slumping and that may be a sign of osteoporosis in your spine. Core stability also helps you to balance and avoid falls and fractures.

5-minute practice

Star breath, in constructive rest pose (savasana) with bellows breath (slow kapalabhati breathing), lying on the mat, 3 rounds of 10 breaths.

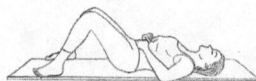

15-minute practice

Bear pose (bhallukasana), for 5–10 breaths.

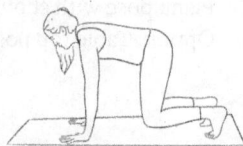

Plank pose (phalankasana). Hold for 10 breaths.

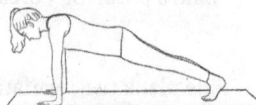

Child's pose (balasana), for 5–10 breaths.

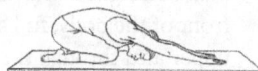

Improving posture (to prevent osteoporotic kyphosis)

5-minute practice

Choose one or two of these poses followed by a counterpose for your spine, e.g., child's pose (balasana) on the mat or a seated forward fold (paschimottanasana), resting your rib cage on your thighs to support your spine.

Standing wall arm raise. Stand against a wall with feet hip distance apart. Zip up the pubic bone to the lower ribs to engage the core abdominal muscles.

Inhale as you slowly raise your right arm, exhale slowly as you lower your right arm. Inhale slowly as you raise your left arm, exhale slowly as you lower your left arm. Repeat 5 times each side.

Tip: If your ribs flare out as you raise your arm, zip up your core and only raise your arm as high as you can maintain control.

Option: Sit upright in a chair with the back of the chair against a wall. Practise these arm raises and notice how close your hand comes to the wall. If you have shoulder pain or frozen shoulder, stand facing the wall with your hands on the wall at shoulder height. Slide your right hand up the wall as you inhale. As you exhale, slide your hand down to shoulder height again. Repeat with your left hand. Practise this for 1–2 minutes, then slide both hands up the wall and down. Notice whether your range of movement has increased.

Mountain pose (tadasana), with a strap. Stand with your feet hip distance apart and place a yoga block midway up your thighs so that you can squeeze it. Hold a yoga strap in your hands, approximately outer hip or shoulder distance apart. Inhale, raise your arms up above your head, and exhale. Take 2–4 breaths with your arms raised and notice if your ribs flare out. Zip up your core and lower your arms to a position where you can maintain this posture. Lower your arms slowly on an exhalation.

Cobra pose (bujangasana) lifts. Raise and lower the chest.

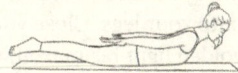

Tip: If you feel discomfort in your lower back, place a folded blanket underneath your hip bones to reduce pressure on the lower back. Exhale as you lift your chest instead of inhaling.

Locust pose A (salabhasana), with arms reaching back.

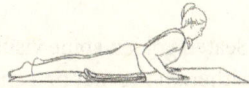

Modifications: Lifting on an inhalation can help you feel a stretch across your chest and collarbone, which can feel energizing and help you breathe more deeply into your lungs. However, if you feel lower back discomfort, try locust pose B: put your hands beside your ribs, place a blanket under your hips and lift on an exhalation to engage your core abdominal muscles. Alternatively, practise locust pose C: hold a yoga strap or belt behind your back approx. hip distance apart, with your knuckles facing the floor.

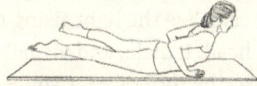

Counterpose: Child's pose (balasana), on the mat or a seated forward fold resting your rib cage on your thighs to support your spine. Stay for 4–6 breaths, and then sit upright and notice your posture. Does your spine feel more upright? How do you feel?

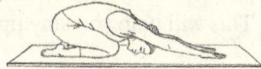

15-minute practice

Arm raises at the wall, 10 times.

Chair pose (modified utkatasana), with a brick
between the thighs.

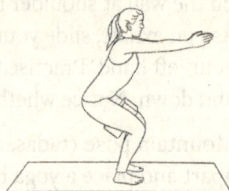

Locust pose (salabasana) or cobra pose
(bujangasana), 10 lifts.

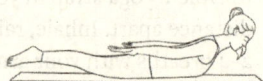

Child's pose (balasana), for 10 breaths.

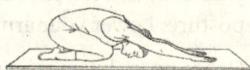

Seated golden spine visualization. Sit upright,
either on the mat or a chair. Root down through
your sit bones and feet to lift and lengthen the
spine upwards. Place two fingers on the crown
of your head (sahasraha chakra), and press down
gently for a few breaths. Then relax your hand
onto your legs. Close your eyes and visualize a
golden light beam from your sit bones up your
spine to the crown of your head. As you inhale,
visualize the light rising to the crown of your
head. Exhale, and visualize the light descending
to the root of your spine (muladhara chakra).
Repeat 10 times, then relax and breathe naturally.

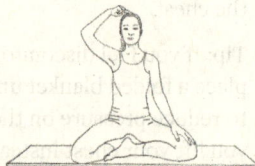

Options: Use imagery that has meaning for you.
Some people prefer the image of a tall tree or a
sunflower reaching towards the sky. Some people
like the image of the crown chakra opening like a
lotus flower.

Modification: Place an upturned bolster along
your spine against a wall or the back of a chair.
This will help you stay upright.

Watch the video on muscle strength.*

MY CLASS FOR HEART HEALTH

Stress is not always a bad thing. Aerobic exercise that carefully raises your heart rate and deepens your breathing is a positive way to keep your heart and lungs healthy. If you carefully challenge these organs with small bursts of exercise, your body will learn to regulate your nervous system when you experience negative stress in your daily life, as well as vasomotor symptoms – hot flushes and heart palpitations, anxiety and panic attacks. Aerobic simply means exercise that increases your heart rate and uses oxygen to produce energy.

Yoga may not be enough to prevent cardiovascular disease, but these static poses held for a minimum of one minute are a good starting point. The slow, mindful breathing practice trains your nervous system to stay calm, even in challenging situations. It is a dress rehearsal for facing stress in your life.

Static held yoga poses carefully raise your heart rate, expand your lungs and tone the muscles around your midriff for weight management, and you can learn to regulate your nervous system with slow breathing.

5-minute practice

Breath of joy, 10 rounds.

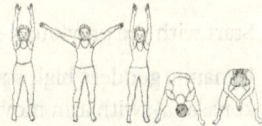

Sun salutation (surya namaskar), 1–4 times.

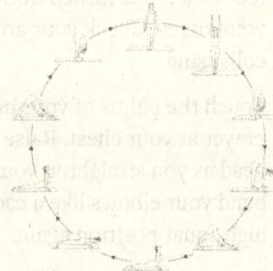

---

* https://www.youtube.com/playlist?list=PLJ-mltZchfBB9d6nOWWnOCaYHP4aQDOWC

Warrior 2 pose (virabhadrasana II), 10 slow breaths with your left leg in front, then your right leg in front for 10 slow breaths.

Benefits: Staying in this pose for a minimum of 10 breaths (1 minute) raises the heart rate, expands the lungs and develops mental resilience and willpower.

Options: If you have a frozen shoulder, place the hand of that arm on your chest so you can feel your breathing and heart rate. If your upper back and neck muscles feel tight, turn the palms of your hands upwards and allow your shoulder blades to slide down away from your ears, and relax.

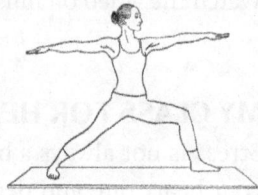

Mountain pose (tadasana), 6–10 breaths. Focus on slowing down your breathing to slow down your heart rate. Use ocean breath (ujjayi pranayama) with your mouth closed and allow your breath to gently stroke the back of your throat. This slight constriction of the throat will slow down your breath and create a calming whisper sound that calms your nervous system.

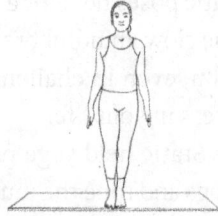

15-minute practice

Start with the previous 5-minute practice, and then add these poses:

Dynamic goddess high squat pose (utkata konasana), with arm movements. Stand with feet wide, toes turned out, heels turned in. Bend your knees. Check your arches are lifted and not collapsing.

Touch the palms of your hands together in a prayer at your chest. Raise your arms above your head as you straighten your legs. Exhale as you bend your elbows like a cactus and return to a high squat position again.

Repeat these arm and leg movements 10 times.

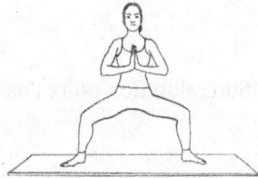

Extended side angle pose (utthita parsvakonasana), on the left side. Stay for 5–10 breaths. Repeat on the right side.

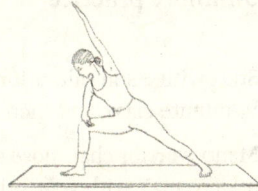

Goddess high squat pose. As above, with 10 small pulses. Start with the palms of your hands in prayer at your chest. Then make small pulsing movements up and down, 10 times.

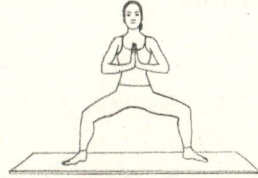

Smaller pulses are more challenging.

Extended triangle pose (uttitha trikonasana), 5–10 breaths on the left side and then change to the right side for 5–10 breaths.

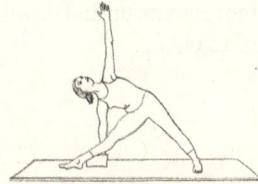

Goddess high squat pose. Start in a high squat with hands in prayer at the front of your heart. Stay here for 10 slow breaths (1 minute).

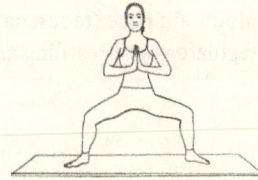

Mountain pose (tadasana).

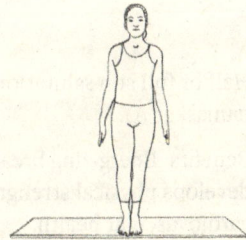

30-minute practice

Start with 4 sun salutations (surya namaskar) followed by the previous 15-minute class, and then add the following:

Meno-warrior chair pose squats (modified utkatasana), with yoga brick or block, 3 x 10 rounds.

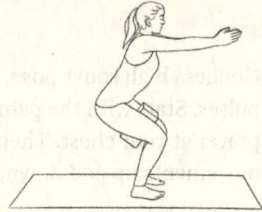

Chair pose (modified utkatasana). Small pulsing movements up and down in the pose for 3 rounds of 10 pulses.

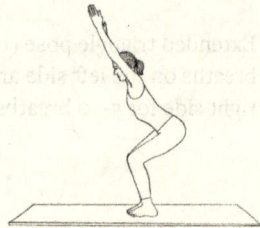

Mountain pose (tadasana), for 5–10 breaths, to regulate your breathing and heart rate.

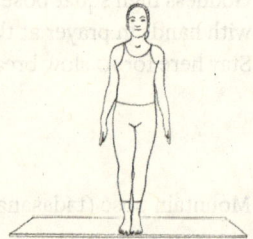

Half or full sun salutation (ardha surya namaskar A).

Benefits: Energizing breath with movement, develops physical strength, flexibility and cardiovascular health.

Beginners: Practise half sun salutation (ardha surya namaskar). Knees on the mat in plank pose (phalakasana) and low crescent lunges (anjaneyasana) instead of the full versions of the poses.

Extended child's pose (utthita balasana) instead of downward facing dog pose (adho mukha svanasana), or have your hands on bricks to make the pose more accessible.

Chair pose (dynamic utkatasana). Swing the arms up and down with the option to lift the heels off the mat.

Beginners and modifications for osteopenia: Squeeze a yoga brick between the thighs to engage your thighs and outer gluteal muscles.

Modification for frozen shoulder: Reach the arms forward and pulse your legs for 10 breaths.

Beginners: Sit on the edge of a chair and then stand up and sit down 10 times.

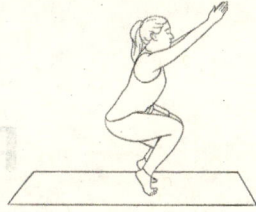

Mountain pose (tadasana), for 5–10 breaths.

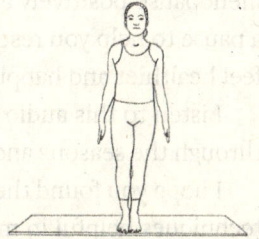

Postscript

Dear friends, I hope this book has helped reframe your view of your menopause positively as your Second Spring, an awakening to yourself, a pause to help you reset and rebalance your life and lifestyle so you can feel healthier and happier in this next liberating stage of your journey.

Listen to this audio recording of my guided visualization taking you through the seasons and stages of life on your journey to Second Spring.

I hope you found the factual information and the yoga techniques helpful in managing some of your symptoms, and feel uplifted and empowered by the reframing of menopause as an opportunity to rebalance your life and lifestyle as you prepare for Second Spring. I hope you found the health and wellbeing advice helpful, and gain some benefits from practising Menopause Yoga daily – even if you only have time for a 5-minute breathing exercise or a meditation or restorative pose, it could make a difference to how you feel.

Your Second Spring may not blossom instantly; like the petals of a precious flower, it may unfold slowly and in stages.

Remember that each woman experiences this journey differently.

Menopause is not an ending, but a beautiful transformation. Embrace this time of self-discovery and create a life that fills you with joy and purpose!

You are not alone! Thank you for joining me on this empowering journey. I hope this book has been a helpful companion.

Watch Petra's final message.

Resources

BOOKS AND ARTICLES

Agombar, F. (2021) *Yoga Therapy for Stress, Burnout and Chronic Fatigue Syndrome*. Jessica Kingsley Publishers.

Anand, A. (2014) *Eat Right for Your Body Type: The Super-Healthy Diet Inspired by Ayurveda*. Quadrille Publishing Ltd.

Baldaniya, H.V. (2017) 'Rajonivruti (Menopause) – Ayurvedic point of view.' *Journal of Ayurveda and Integrated Medical Sciences 2*, 1. https://doi.org/10.21760/jaims.v2i1.7503

Bammel Wilding, A. (2017) *Wild & Wise: Sacred Feminine Meditations for Women's Circles & Personal Awakening*. Womancraft Publishing.

Clennell, B. (2007) *The Woman's Yoga Book: Asana and Pranayama for all Phases of the Menstrual Cycle*. Shambhala Publications.

Codrington, K. (2024) *The Perimenopause Journal*. David & Charles.

Dinsmore-Tuli, U. (2019) *Yoni Shakti: A Woman's Guide to Power and Freedom Through Yoga and Tantra*. Yoga Words, an imprint of Pinter & Martin Ltd.

Emerson, D. (2015) *Trauma-Sensitive Yoga in Therapy: Bringing the Body into Treatment*. W.W. Norton & Company.

Emerson, D. and Hopper, E. (2011) *Overcoming Trauma Through Yoga: Reclaiming Your Body*. North Atlantic Books.

Francina, S. (2015) *Yoga and the Wisdom of Menopause: A Guide to Physical, Emotional and Spiritual Health at Midlife and Beyond*. Health Communications, Inc.

Frawley, D. (2000) *Ayurvedic Healing: A Comprehensive Guide*. Lotus Press.

Frawley, D. (2009) *Yoga & Ayurveda: Self Healing and Self-Realization*. Lotus Press.

Frawley, D. and Lad, V. (1994) *The Yoga of Herbs: An Ayurvedic Guide to Herbal Medicine*. Lotus Press.

Fugate Woods, N., Sullivan Mitchell, E., Percival, D.B. and Smith-DiJulio, K. (2009) 'Is the menopausal transition painful? Observations of perceived stress from the Seattle Midlife Women's Health Study.' *Menopause 16*, 1, 90–97. doi: 10.1097/gme.0b013e31817ed261.

Greer, G. (1991) *The Change: Women, Aging and the Menopause*. Ballantine Books.

Hanson Lasater, J. (2011) *Relax and Renew: Restful Yoga for Stressful Times*. Shambhala Publications.

Hillard, T., Abernethy, K., Hamoda, H., Shaw, I., *et al.* (2017) *Management of the Menopause*. Sixth edn. British Menopause Society.

Hope, A. (2016) *Holding Space: A Guide to Supporting Others While Remembering to Take Care of Yourself First*. All Things That Matter Press.

Iyengar, G.S. (2013) *Yoga: A Gem for Women*. Allied Publishers Pvt. Ltd.

Lad, V. (2002) *Textbook of Ayurveda: Fundamental Principles*, Vol. 1. The Ayurvedic Press.

Lad, V. (2006) *Textbook of Ayurveda: A Complete Guide to Clinical Practice*, Vol. 2. The Ayurvedic Press.

Lad, V. (2012) *Textbook of Ayurveda: General Principles of Management and Treatment*, Vol. 3. The Ayurvedic Press.

Levine, P. (1997) *Waking the Tiger: Healing Trauma*. North Atlantic Books.

Levine, P. (2017) *In an Unspoken Voice: How the Body Releases Trauma and Restores Goodness*. North Atlantic Books.

McCall, T. (2007) *Yoga as Medicine: The Yogic Prescription for Health and Healing*. Bantam Dell, a Division of Random House, Inc.

McIntyre, A. and Boudin, M. (2012) *Dispensing with Tradition: A Practitioner's Guide to Using Indian and Western Herbs the Ayurvedic Way*. Artemis House.

Mehta, L. (2024) *The Feel Good Fix: Boost Energy, Improve Sleep and Move More Through Menopause and Beyond*. Penguin.

Mosconi, L. (2024) *The Menopause Brain: The New Science Empowering Women to Navigate Midlife with Knowledge and Confidence*. Atlantic Books.

Newby, K. (2024) *The Natural Menopause Method: A Nutritional Guide to Perimenopause and Beyond*. Pavilion Books.

Panda, G.K., Arya, B.C., Sharma, M.K. and Rani, M. (2018) 'Menopausal syndrome and its management with Ayurveda.' *Internal Journal of Health Sciences and Research 8*, 5, 337–341. www.ijhsr.org/IJHSR_Vol.8_Issue.5_May2018/48.pdf

Pope, A. and Wurlitzer, S.H. (2017) *Wild Power: Discover the Magic of Your Menstrual Cycle and Awaken the Feminine Path to Power*. Hay House.

Porges, S. (2017) *The Pocket Guide to the Polyvagal Theory: The Transformative Power of Feeling Safe*. W.W. Norton & Company.

Powers, S. (2008) *Insight Yoga: An Innovative Synthesis of Traditional Yoga, Meditation, and Eastern Approaches to Healing and Wellbeing*. Shambhala Publications.

Rothschild, B. (2000) *The Body Remembers: The Psychophysiology of Trauma and Trauma Treatment*. W.W. Norton & Company.

Satyananda Saraswati, S. (2013) *Asana Pranayama Mudra Bandha*. Bihar School of Yoga.

Sharan, F. (1994) *Creative Menopause*. Wisdom Press.

Sharma, R.K. and Dash, B. (2008) *Caraka Samhita: Volumes I, II & III*. Chowkhamba Sanskrit Series Office. www.narayana-verlag.com/homeopathy/pdf/Caraka-Samhita-7-Volumes-R-K-Sharma-Vaidya-Bhagwan-Dash.07927_1Contents_Volume_1.pdf

Siegel, D. (2011) *Mindsight: The New Science of Personal Transformation*. Oneworld Publications.

Siegel, D. (2012) *Pocket Guide to Interpersonal Neurobiology: An Integrative Handbook of the Mind*. W.W. Norton & Company.

Strom, M. (2013) *There Is No App for Happiness: Finding Joy and Meaning in the Digital Age with Mindfulness, Breathwork, and Yoga*. Skyhorse Publishing.

Svoboda, R.E. (1999) *Ayurveda for Women: A Guide to Vitality and Health*. Healing Arts Press.

Swan, N. (2002) 'The HRT scare.' ABC Health & Wellbeing, 6 August. www.abc.net.au/health/minutes/stories/2002/08/06/641540.htm

Tiwari, M. (2007) *Women's Power to Heal Through Inner Medicine*. Mother Om Media.

van der Kolk, B. (2015) *The Body Keeps the Score: Brain and Body in the Transformation of Trauma*. Penguin.

Walters, V. (1993) 'Stress, anxiety and depression: Women's accounts of their health problems.' *Social Science & Medicine 36*, 4, 393–402. doi: 10.1016/0277-9536(93)90401-0.

Watts, C. (2018) *Yoga Therapy For Digestive Health*. Singing Dragon.

Weed, S.S. (2002) *New Menopausal Years: The Wise Woman Way*. Ash Tree Publishing.

WEBSITES

A4TE (Advocate for Trans Equality): www.transequality.org

Age UK: www.ageuk.org.uk/information-advice/health-wellbeing/conditions-illnesses/osteoporosis

BHOF (Bone Health and Osteoporosis Foundation): www.bonehealthandosteoporosis.org/patients/patient-support/faq

British Menopause Society: https://thebms.org.uk

Charlotte Watts: www.charlottewattshealth.com

Daisy Network: www.daisynetwork.org/about-poi/what-is-poi

Emma's Nutrition: www.emmasnutrition.com

Harmonise You, women's health practitioner: https://harmoniseyou.co.uk

International Menopause Society: www.imsociety.org

Jinty Sheerin's WomenKind Collective podcast: https://shows.acast.com/womenkind-collective

Karen Arthur's 'Menopause Whilst Black' podcast: www.menopausewhilstblack.com

Look Good Feel Better Foundation, body confidence and self-esteem: https://lookgoodfeelbetter.org/programs/around-the-world

Maggie's support centres and online information: www.maggies.org

Menopause and Cancer Podcast: https://menopauseandcancer.org/podcast

National Autistic Society, autism and the menopause: www.autism.org.uk/advice-and-guidance/topics/physical-health/menopause#Autism%20and%20the%20menopause

NHS: www.nhs.uk/conditions/osteoporosis/living-with; www.nhs.uk/conditions/early-menopause

Royal Osteoporosis Society: https://theros.org.uk

The Menopause Society™ (formerly North American Menopause Society™): www.menopause.org

Women's Health Concern: www.womens-health-concern.org/help-and-advice/factsheets/menopause

Yoga for Cancer Academy, free yoga videos for home practice: www.youtube.com/@YogaForCancerAcademy

Yoga for Cancer Teacher Register: www.yogaforcanceracademy.org/yfca-teacher-register

Endnotes

Preface

1   Zhao, X. (2006) *Traditional Chinese Medicine for Women: Reflections of the Moon on Water*. Virago.

Introduction

1   NICE (National Institute for Health and Care Excellence) (2015) *Menopause: Identification and Management*. NICE guideline 23 (NG23), Section 1.1 [last updated 7 November 2024]. www.nice.org.uk/guidance/ng23/chapter/Recommendations#individualised-care

Part 1

1   Wilson, R.A. (1966) *Feminine Forever*. M. Evans and Company, Inc.

2   Kohn, G.E., Rodriguez, K.M., Hotaling, J. and Pastuszak, A.W. (2019) 'The history of estrogen therapy.' *Sexual Medicine Reviews* 7, 3, 416–421. doi: 10.1016/j.sxmr.2019.03.006.

3   Pahwa, R., Goyal, A. and Jialal, I. (2023) 'Chronic inflammation.' StatPearls Publishing [updated 7 August 2023]. www.ncbi.nlm.nih.gov/books/NBK493173

4   McEwen, B.S. (1998) 'Stress, adaptation, and disease. Allostasis and allostatic load.' *Annals of the New York Academy of Sciences* 840, 33–44. doi: 10.1111/j.1749-6632.1998.tb09546.x.

5   British Heart Foundation (no date) 'Menopause and your heart.' www.bhf.org.uk/informationsupport/support/women-with-a-heart-condition/menopause-and-heart-disease

6   Klop, C., van Staa, T.P., Cooper, C., Harvey, N.C. and de Vries, F. (2017) 'The epidemiology of mortality after fracture in England: Variation by age, sex, time, geographic location, and ethnicity.' *Osteoporosis International* 28, 161–168. https://doi.org/10.1007/s00198-016-3787-0

7   Boulin, T., Whitcroft, I. and Moody, H. (2024) 'HRT, menopause and breast cancer.' Breast Cancer UK. https://cdn.breastcanceruk.org.uk/uploads/2024/02/HRT-and-Breast-Cancer-Review-Breast-Cancer-UK-1.pdf

8   Patchev, V.K. and Patchev, A.V. (2006) 'Experimental models of stress.' *Dialogues in Clinical Neuroscience* 8, 4, 417–432. www.ncbi.nlm.nih.gov/pmc/articles/PMC3181831

9   Messier, V., Rabasa-Lhoret, R., Barbat-Artigas, S., Elisha, B., Karelis, A.D. and Aubertin-Leheudre, M. (2011) 'Menopause and sarcopenia: A potential role for sex hormones.' *Maturitas* 68, 4, 331–336. doi: 10.1016/j.maturitas.2011.01.014. https://pubmed.ncbi.nlm.nih.gov/21353405; Walston, J.D. (2012) 'Sarcopenia in older adults.' *Current Opinion in Rheumatology* 24, 6, 623–627. doi: 10.1097/BOR.0b013e328358d59b. www.ncbi.nlm.nih.gov/pmc/articles/PMC4066461

10 Tran, Q. (2022) 'Leading charity urges action as analysis shows dementia has been UK women's leading cause of death for a decade.' Alzheimer's Research UK News, 15 May. www.alzheimersresearchuk.org/news/leading-charity-urges-action-as-analysis-shows-dementia-has-been-uk-womens-leading-cause-of-death-for-a-decade

11 Mosconi, L. (2024) *The Menopause Brain: The New Science Empowering Women to Navigate Midlife with Knowledge and Confidence.* Atlantic Books, p.6.

12 NICE (National Institute for Health and Care Excellence) (2015) *Menopause: Identification and Management.* NICE guideline 23 (NG23), Section 1.1 [last updated 7 November 2024]. www.nice.org.uk/guidance/ng23/chapter/Recommendations#individualised-care

13 Daisy Network (no date) 'What is POI' www.daisynetwork.org/about-poi/what-is-poi

14 NHS (no date) 'Early or premature menopause.' [Last reviewed 11 March 2025.] www.nhs.uk/conditions/early-or-premature-menopause

15 WHO (World Health Organization) (2024) 'Post-traumatic stress disorder.' Fact sheet, 27 May. www.who.int/news-room/fact-sheets/detail/post-traumatic-stress-disorder

16 Khouri, H. (2021) *Peace from Anxiety: Get Grounded, Build Resilience, and Stay Connected Amidst the Chaos.* Shambhala Publications, p.18.

17 Ibid, p.91.

18 Pinkerton, J.V., Doughterty, P. and Modesitt, S.C. (2008) 'The effects of abuse on health problems in menopausal women.' *Menopause* 15, 1, 1–4. doi: 10.1097/gme.0b013e31815b89ec. https://pubmed.ncbi.nlm.nih.gov/18090873/2018

19 Gibson, C.J., Huang, A.J., McCaw, B., Subak, L.L., Thom, D.H. and van den Eeden, S.K. (2019) 'Associations of intimate partner violence, sexual assault, and posttraumatic stress disorder with menopause symptoms among midlife and older women.' *JAMA Internal Medicine* 179, 1, 80–87. doi: 10.1001/jamainternmed.2018.5233. https://jamanetwork.com/journals/jamainternalmedicine/fullarticle/2715160

20 Fawcett Society (2022) 'Landmark study: Menopausal women let down by employers and healthcare providers.' News & Views, 2 May. www.fawcettsociety.org.uk/news/landmark-study-menopausal-women-let-down-by-employers-and-healthcare-providers

21 Pfaltz, M.C. and Schnyder, U. (2023) 'Allostatic load and allostatic overload: Preventive and clinical implications.' *Psychotherapy and Psychosomatics* 92, 5, 279–282. doi: 10.1159/000534340. www.ncbi.nlm.nih.gov/pmc/articles/PMC10716872

22 McEwen, B.S. and Stellar, E. (1993) 'Stress and the individual: Mechanisms leading to disease.' *Archives of Internal Medicine* 153, 18, 2093–2101. doi: 10.1001/

archinte.1993.00410180039004; Hillman, S., Shantikumar, S., Ridha, A., Todkill, D. and Dale, J. (2020) 'Socioeconomic status and HRT prescribing: A study of practice-level data in England.' *British Journal of General Practice* 70, 700, e772–e777. https://doi.org/10.3399/bjgp20X713045

23 Quoted from Karen Arthur's 'Menopause Whilst Black' podcast: www.menopausewhilstblack.com

24 BMS (British Menopause Society) (2022) 'Induced menopause in women with endometriosis.' Tool for clinicians. https://thebms.org.uk/wp-content/uploads/2022/12/10-BMS-TfC-Induced-Menopause-in-women-with-endometriosis-NOV2022-A.pdf

25 BMS (British Menopause Society) (2022–2024) 'Surgical menopause: A toolkit for healthcare professionals.' Tool for clinicians. https://thebms.org.uk/wp-content/uploads/2023/01/13-BMS-TfC-Surgical-Menopause-JAN2023-A.pdf

26 Hickey, M., Basu, P., Sassarini, J., Stegmann, M.E., *et al.* (2024) 'Managing menopause after cancer.' *The Lancet* 403, 10430, 984–996. doi: 10.1016/S0140-6736(23)02802-7.

27 BMS (British Menopause Society) (2022) 'NICE: Menopause, diagnosis and management – from guideline to practice.' Guideline Summary. https://thebms.org.uk/wp-content/uploads/2016/04/NICE-Menopause-Diagnosis-and-Management-from-Guideline-to-Practice-Guideline-Summary.pdf

28 Guidi, J., Lucente, M., Sonino, N. and Fava, G.A. (2021) 'Allostatic load and its impact on health: A systematic review.' *Psychotherapy and Psychosomatics* 90, 1, 11–27. doi: 10.1159/000510696.

29 Glyde, T. (2021) 'How can therapists and other healthcare practitioners best support and validate their queer menopausal clients?' *Sexual and Relationship Therapy* 38, 4, 1–24, pp.5–6. https://doi.org/10.1080/14681994.2021.1881770

30 Duffy, S. (2024) 'Grounding in Groundlessness, Being the Change: An existential phenomenological exploration into the embodied experience of postmenopause.' DProf thesis, Middlesex University London. https://repository.mdx.ac.uk/item/148z12

31 Glyde, T. (2021) 'How can therapists and other healthcare practitioners best support and validate their queer menopausal clients?' *Sexual and Relationship Therapy* 38, 4, 1–24. https://doi.org/10.1080/14681994.2021.1881770; Glyde, T. (2022) 'LGBTQIA+ menopause: Room for improvement.' *The Lancet* 400, 10363, 1578–1579. https://doi.org/10.1016/S0140-6736(22)01935-3

32 Dillaway, H.E. (2005) '(Un)changing menopausal bodies: How women think and act in the face of a reproductive transition and gendered beauty ideals. *Sex Roles* 53, 1–2, 1–17. https://doi.org/10.1007/s11199-005-4269-6; Ussher, J.M. (2006) *Managing the Monstrous Feminine: Regulating the Reproductive Body.* Routledge.

33 Winterich, J.A. (2003) 'Sex, menopause, and culture: Sexual orientation and the meaning of menopause for women's sex lives.' *Gender & Society* 17, 4, 627–642. https://doi.org/10.1177/0891243203253962

34 Study of Women's Health Across the Nation (SWAN): www.swanstudy.org

35 Mosconi, L. (2024) *The Menopause Brain: The New Science Empowering Women to Navigate Midlife with Knowledge and Confidence.* Atlantic Books, pp.93–94.

36 Ibid, p.93.

Part 2

1   BBC Radio 4 (2024) 'Just one thing – with Michael Mosley.' www.bbc.co.uk/programmes/p09by3yy/episodes/downloads

2   Bommer, S., Klein, P. and Suter, A. (2011) 'First time proof of sage's tolerability and efficacy in menopausal women with hot flushes.' *Advances in Therapy* 28, 6, 490–500. https://doi.org/10.1007/s12325-011-0027-z; Briese, V., Stammwitz, U., Friede, M. and Henneicke-von Zepelin, H.-H. (2007) 'Black cohosh with or without St. John's wort for symptom-specific climacteric treatment – Results of a large-scale, controlled, observational study.' *Maturitas* 57, 4, 405–414. https://doi.org/10.1016/j.maturitas.2007.04.008; Castelo-Branco, C., Gambacciani, M., Cano, A., Minkin, M.J., *et al.* (2020) 'Review & meta-analysis: Isopropanolic black cohosh extract iCR for menopausal symptoms – An update on the evidence.' *Climacteric* 24, 2, 1–11. https://doi.org/10.1080/13697137.2020.18 20477; Gerbarg, P.L. and Brown, R.P. (2016) 'Pause menopause with Rhodiola rosea, a natural selective estrogen receptor modulator.' *Phytomedicine* 23, 7, 763–769. https://doi.org/10.1016/j.phymed.2015.11.013

3   Soules, M.R., Sherman, S., Parrott, E., Rebar, R., *et al.* (2001) 'Executive summary: Stages of Reproductive Aging Workshop (STRAW).' *Climacteric* 4, 267–272. www.imsociety.org/wp-content/uploads/2020/08/statement-2001-07-23.pdf

4   Watson, S.L., Weeks, B.K., Weis, L.J., Harding, A.T., Horan, S.A. and Beck, B.R. (2017) 'High-intensity resistance and impact training improves bone mineral density and physical function in postmenopausal women with osteopenia and osteoporosis: The LIFTMOR randomized controlled trial.' *Journal of Bone and Mineral Research* 33, 2, 211–220. doi: 10.1002/jbmr.3284.

5   Mehta, L. (2024) *The Feel Good Fix: Boost Energy, Improve Sleep and Move More Through Menopause and Beyond.* Penguin, p.63.

6   Ewert, A. and Chang, Y. (2018) 'Levels of nature and stress response.' *Behavioral Sciences (Basel)* 8, 5, 49. doi: 10.3390/bs8050049. www.ncbi.nlm.nih.gov/pmc/articles/PMC5981243

7   Pound, M., Massey, H., Roseneil, S., Williamson, R., *et al.* (2024) 'How do women feel cold water swimming affects their menstrual and perimenopausal symptoms?' *Post Reproductive Health* 30, 1. https://doi.org/10.1177/20533691241227100

8   UCL (2024) 'Cold water swimming improves menopause symptoms.' UCL News, 25 January. www.ucl.ac.uk/news/2024/jan/cold-water-swimming-improves-menopause-symptoms

9   Islam H, Gibala MJ, Little JP. Exercise Snacks: A Novel Strategy to Improve Cardiometabolic Health. Exerc Sport Sci Rev. 2022 Jan 1;50(1):31-37. doi: 10.1249/JES.0000000000000275. PMID: 34669625.

Part 3

1   Bisht, S., Banu, S., Srivastava, S., Pathak, R.U., *et al.* (2020) 'Sperm methylome alterations following yoga-based lifestyle intervention in patients of primary male infertility: A pilot study.' *Andrologia 52*, 4, e13551. https://doi.org/10.1111/and.13551; Dada, R., Gautam, S., Dada, T., Tiwari, P. and Kumar, M. (2023) 'Yoga: Unraveling the internal pharmacy – impact on genome and epigenome.' *Medical Research Archives 11*, 12. doi: 10.18103/mra.v11i12.4877; Kumari, D., Kumar, M., Tiwari, P., Mahey, R., *et al.* (2023) 'Impact of Yoga in polycystic ovary syndrome.' *International Journal of Ayurveda Research 4*, 3, 132–136. doi: 10.4103/ijar.ijar_133_23; Dada, T., Bhai, N., Midha, N., Shakrawal, J., *et al.* (2021) 'Effect of mindfulness meditation on intraocular pressure and trabecular meshwork gene expression: A randomized controlled trial.' *American Journal of Ophthalmology 223*, 308–321. doi: 10.1016/j.ajo.2020.10.012; Dada, T., Mondal, S., Midha, N., Mahalingam, K., *et al.* (2022) 'Effect of mindfulness-based stress reduction on intraocular pressure in patients with ocular hypertension: A randomized control trial.' *American Journal of Ophthalmology 239*, 66–73. doi: 10.1016/j.ajo.2022.01.017; Dhawan, V., Kumar, M., Deka, D., Malhotra, N., *et al.* (2018) 'Meditation & yoga: Impact on oxidative DNA damage & dysregulated sperm transcripts in male partners of couples with recurrent pregnancy loss.' *Indian Journal of Medical Research 148*, Suppl. 1, S134–S139. doi: 10.4103/ijmr. IJMR_1988_17; Dhawan, V., Malhotra, N., Singh, N., Dadhwal, V. and Dada, R. (2024) 'Yoga and its effect on sperm genomic integrity, gene expression, telomere length and perceived quality of life in early pregnancy loss.' *Scientific Reports 14*, 1, 11711. doi: 10.1038/s41598-024-62380-w; Gautam, S., Kumar, M., Kumar, U. and Dada, R. (2020) 'Effect of an 8-week yoga-based lifestyle intervention on psycho-neuro-immune axis, disease activity, and perceived quality of life in rheumatoid arthritis patients: A randomized controlled trial.' *Frontiers in Psychology 11*, 2259. https://doi.org/10.3389/fpsyg.2020.02259; Gautam, S., Kumar, R., Kumar, U., Kumar, S., Luthra, K. and Dada, R. (2023) 'Yoga maintains Th17/Treg cell homeostasis and reduces the rate of T cell aging in rheumatoid arthritis: A randomized controlled trial.' *Scientific Reports 13*, 1, 14924. doi: 10.1038/s41598-023-42231-w; Gautam, S., Kumar, U., Kumar, M., Rana, D. and Dada, R. (2021) 'Yoga improves mitochondrial health and reduces severity of autoimmune inflammatory arthritis: A randomized controlled trial.' *Mitochondrion 58*, 147–159. doi: 10.1016/j.mito.2021.03.004; Tolahunase, M.R., Sagar, R. and Dada, R. (2018) '5-HTTLPR and MTHFR 677C>T polymorphisms and response to yoga-based lifestyle intervention in major depressive disorder: A randomized active-controlled trial.' *Indian Journal of Psychiatry 60*, 4, 410–426. doi: 10.4103/psychiatry.IndianJPsychiatry_398_17.

2   Dada, T., Bhai, N., Midha, N., Shakrawal, J., *et al.* (2021) 'Effect of mindfulness meditation on intraocular pressure and trabecular meshwork gene expression: A randomized controlled trial.' *American Journal of Ophthalmology 223*, 308–321. doi: 10.1016/j.ajo.2020.10.012; Dada, T., Mondal, S., Midha, N., Mahalingam, K., *et al.* (2022) 'Effect of mindfulness-based stress reduction on intraocular pressure in patients with ocular hypertension: A randomized

control trial.' *American Journal of Ophthalmology* 239, 66–73. doi: 10.1016/j. ajo.2022.01.017; Dada, R., Gautam, S., Dada, T., Tiwari, P. and Kumar, M. (2023) 'Yoga: Unraveling the internal pharmacy – impact on genome and epigenome.' *Medical Research Archives* 11, 12. doi: 10.18103/mra.v11i12.4877; Gautam, S., Kumar, M., Kumar, U. and Dada, R. (2020) 'Effect of an 8-week yoga-based lifestyle intervention on psycho-neuro-immune axis, disease activity, and perceived quality of life in rheumatoid arthritis patients: A randomized controlled trial.' *Frontiers in Psychology* 11, 2259. https://doi. org/10.3389/fpsyg.2020.02259; Gautam, S., Kumar, R., Kumar, U., Kumar, S., Luthra, K. and Dada, R. (2023) 'Yoga maintains Th17/Treg cell homeostasis and reduces the rate of T cell aging in rheumatoid arthritis: A randomized controlled trial.' *Scientific Reports* 13, 1, 14924. doi: 10.1038/s41598-023-42231-w.

3   Tolahunase, M.R., Sagar, R. and Dada, R. (2018) '5-HTTLPR and MTHFR 677C>T polymorphisms and response to yoga-based lifestyle intervention in major depressive disorder: A randomized active-controlled trial.' *Indian Journal of Psychiatry* 60, 4, 410–426. doi: 10.4103/psychiatry. IndianJPsychiatry_398_17.

4   Gautam, S., Kumar, M., Kumar, U. and Dada, R. (2020) 'Effect of an 8-week yoga-based lifestyle intervention on psycho-neuro-immune axis, disease activity, and perceived quality of life in rheumatoid arthritis patients: A randomized controlled trial.' *Frontiers in Psychology* 11, 2259. https://doi. org/10.3389/fpsyg.2020.02259

5   Mastrangelo, M.A., Galantino, M.L. and House, L. (2007) 'Effects of yoga on quality of life and flexibility in menopausal women: A case series.' *Explore (New York, NY)* 3, 1, 42–45. doi: 10.1016/j.explore.2006.10.007

Part 4

1   Welch, C. (2011) *Balance Your Hormones, Balance Your Life: Achieving Optimal Health and Wellness Through Ayurveda, Chinese Medicine, and Western Science.* Da Capo Lifelong Books (see pp.1–2).

2   Mosconi, L. (2024) *The New Science Empowering Women to Navigate Midlife with Knowledge and Confidence.* Atlantic Books, p.93.

3   Strom, M. (2010) *A Life Worth Breathing: A Yoga Master's Handbook of Strength, Grace, and Healing.* Skyhorse Publishing.

4   Traister, R. (2018) *Good and Mad: The Revolutionary Power of Women's Anger.* Simon & Schuster.

5   Hunter, M. and Smith, M. (2014) *Managing Hot Flushes and Night Sweats: A Cognitive Behavioural Self-Help Guide to the Menopause.* Routledge. See also Carmody, J.F., Crawford, S., Salmoirago-Blotcher, E., Leung, K., Churchill, L. and Olendzki, N. (2011) 'Mindfulness training for coping with hot flushes: Results of a randomized trial.' *Menopause (New York, NY)* 18, 6, 611–620. doi: 10.1097/gme.0b013e318204a05c.

6   Hunter, M. and Smith, M. (2014) *Managing Hot Flushes and Night Sweats: A Cognitive Behavioural Self-Help Guide to the Menopause*. Routledge (see pages 35–40 and 47–48 in particular).

7   Crider, C. (2024) 'Why does joint pain get worse around menopause?' Healthline, 18 April. www.healthline.com/health/menopause/joint-pain-menopause

8   Rath, J. (2022) 'What is arthritis?' Arthritis Foundation, 9 June. www.arthritis.org/health-wellness/about-arthritis/understanding-arthritis/what-is-arthritis

9   The Menopause Charity (no date) 'Joint pain and muscles.' www.themenopausecharity.org/2021/10/21/joint-pain-and-muscles; NIH (National Institutes of Health) (2022) 'Magnesium.' Fact sheets https://ods.od.nih.gov/factsheets/Magnesium-HealthProfessional

10   Scheiber, A. and Mank, V. (2023) 'Anti-inflammatory diets.' StatPearls Publishing. www.ncbi.nlm.nih.gov/books/NBK597377

11   Kozinoga, M., Majchrzycki, M. and Piotrowska, S. (2015) 'Low back pain in women before and after menopause.' *Przeglad Menopauzalny* 14, 3, 203–207. doi: 10.5114/pm.2015.54347.

12   NHS (no date) 'Exercises for sciatica problems.' www.nhs.uk/live-well/exercise/exercises-sciatica-problems

13   Al-Subahi, M., Alayat, M., Alshehri, M.A., Helal, O., *et al.* (2017) 'The effectiveness of physiotherapy interventions for sacroiliac joint dysfunction: A systematic review.' *Journal of Physical Therapy Science* 29, 9, 1689–1694. doi: 10.1589/jpts.29.1689.

14   NHS (no date) 'Exercises for sciatica problems.' www.nhs.uk/live-well/exercise/exercises-sciatica-problems

15   Sanfilippo, L. (2019) *Yoga Therapy for Insomnia and Sleep Recovery*. Singing Dragon.

16   Hunter, M. and Smith, M. (2020) *Managing Hot Flushes and Night Sweats: A Cognitive Behavioural Approach to Menopause*. Second edn. Routledge.

17   Sanfilippo, L. (2020) *Sleep Recovery: The Five Step Yoga Solution to Restore Your Rest*. Green Tree, p.112.

18   Stamatakis, E., Ahmadi, M., Biswas, R.K., Del Pozo Cruz, B., *et al.* (2024) 'Device-measured vigorous intermittent lifestyle physical activity (VILPA) and major adverse cardiovascular events: Evidence of sex differences.' *British Journal of Sports Medicine* [online first, 28 October]. doi: 10.1136/bjsports-2024-108484.

19   Ahmadi, M.N., Hamer, M., Gill, J.M.R., Murphy, M., *et al.* (2023) 'Brief bouts of device-measured intermittent lifestyle physical activity and its association with major adverse cardiovascular events and mortality in people who do not exercise: A prospective cohort study.' *The Lancet* 8, 10, E800–E810. www.thelancet.com/journals/lanpub/article/PIIS2468-2667(23)00183-4/fulltext; see also Loughborough University Media Centre, 'Short bursts of daily activity linked to reduced cancer risk' [press release, 28 July]. www.lboro.ac.uk/media-centre/press-releases/2023/july/daily-activity-linked-to-reduced-cancer-risk

20 Wang, T., Laher, I. and Li, S. (2025) 'Exercise snacks and physical fitness in sedentary populations.' *Sports Medicine and Health Science* 7, 1, 1–7. https://doi. org/10.1016/j.smhs.2024.02.006

21 Nourkhalaj, Y. (2024) 'What are exercise snacks and why are they important?' Stanford Lifestyle Medicine, 2 July. https://longevity.stanford.edu/ lifestyle/2024/07/02/what-are-exercise-snacks-and-why-are-they-important

22 Metha, L. (2024) *The Feel Good Fix: Boost Energy, Improve Sleep and Move More Through Menopause and Beyond*. Penguin, p.14.

23 Faubion, S.S., Shuster, L.T. and Bharucha, A.E. (2012) 'Recognition and management of nonrelaxing pelvic floor dysfunction.' *Mayo Clinic Proceedings* 87, 2, 187–193. doi: 10.1016/j.mayocp.2011.09.004.

24 Calais-Germain, B. (2003) *The Female Pelvis: Anatomy & Exercises*; for online female-focused wellness professional education, see Burrell Education, at www.burrelleducation.com; for a somatic approach to psoas and pelvic health, see Core Awareness™ with Liz Koch, at www.coreawareness.com

25 Langhorne, O., Standeven, L. and Thomas, K. (no date) 'Sex after menopause.' Johns Hopkins Medicine. www.hopkinsmedicine.org/health/ wellness-and-prevention/how-sex-changes-after-menopause

26 Hart, J. (no date) 'The surprising effects of stress on your bladder.' National Association for Continence. https://nafc.org/bhealth-blog/ the-surprising-effects-of-stress-on-your-bladder

27 Effects of yoga interventions on the fatigue-pain-sleep disturbance symptom cluster in breast cancer patients: A systematic review Author links open overlay panelYishu Qi, Huiyuan Li, Dorothy Ngo Sheung Chan, Xing Ma, Cho Lee Wong https://www.sciencedirect.com/science/article/abs/pii/ S1462388924000929

28 Breast Cancer UK (no date) 'Exercise: Physical activity and breast cancer.' www. breastcanceruk.org.uk/reduce-your-risk/physical-activity-and-breast-cancer

29 Severinsen, M.C.K. and Pedersen, B.K. (2020) 'Muscle-organ crosstalk: The emerging roles of myokines.' *Endocrine Reviews* 41, 4, 594–609. doi: 10.1210/ endrev/bnaa016. [Erratum in *Endocrine Reviews*, 28 January 2021, 42, 1, 97–99. doi: 10.1210/endrev/bnaa024.]

30 Metha, L. (2024) *The Feel Good Fix: Boost Energy, Improve Sleep and Move More Through Menopause and Beyond*. Penguin, pp.70–71.

31 Cho, E.-J., Choi, Y., Jung, S.-J. and Kwak, H.-B. (2022) 'Role of exercise in oestrogen deficiency-induced sarcopenia.' *Journal of Exercise Rehabilitation* 18, 2–9. https://doi.org/10.12965/jer.2244004.002